# Anger Management Workbook

*Step by Step Guide on How to Manage and Recognize Anger With Specific Techniques*

Steven J. Garratt

Copyright © 2020 Steven J. Garratt

All rights reserved.

# CONTENTS

Introduction .................................................................................... 7

Identifying Your Anger .................................................................. 9

Common Questions About Anger ............................................... 19

What Triggers Your Anger? ......................................................... 29

In What Ways Is Anger a Problem? ............................................ 39

Control Anger Before It Controls You ........................................ 49

CBT for Anger Management ....................................................... 59

Cognitive Distortions That Fuel Anger and How to Deal With Them? .... 71

How to Communicate When You Are Angry? ........................... 81

Tips For Managing Conflicts For People With Anger Issues .......... 91

Reasons Behind Passive-Aggressiveness and Coping Mechanisms ....... 101

Conclusion .................................................................................. 111

# Introduction

Congratulations on purchasing *Anger Management Workbook,* and thank you for doing so.

Just like happiness and sadness, anger is an emotion that we all have to deal with from time to time. In fact, among all emotions, anger is one of the firsts to be experienced by a kid, and so, anger management should be practiced from a young age. It is through anger management that you learn how to balance your feelings, and also teaches you how to view the world. Your own anger, when not kept under control, can make you feel like a victim. Always remember that just like you choose your lunch or dinner, you can choose how to respond to others and whether or not you want to keep your anger under control.

Everyone's root cause for problematic anger is different, and in this book, we will explore different options. People often think that if they do not want others to bully them, they have to reply with their anger, but it doesn't happen like that. There are other ways of responding to others. If you don't deal with your anger issues, it will be like living in a prison of your own making. So, don't delay and start taking action right now!

There are plenty of books on this subject on the market, thanks again for choosing this one! Every effort was made to ensure it is full of as much useful information as possible; please enjoy!

# 1.
# Identifying Your Anger

In this chapter, you are going to get a basic overview of what anger is and the basic aspects of recognizing it because that is the first step of anger management.

## What is Anger?

Anger is a common and natural emotion that is experienced by everyone. It is often irrational and unwanted. Experts describe anger as a way to survive or protect yourself from anything which is considered wrong. Irritation, stress, and tiredness can bring mild anger. People are likely to feel irritated f their basic needs such as sleep, sex, shelter, food, etc. are not met adequately. People often become angry while reacting to a threat, criticism, or frustration. In situations like these, anger is not always an inappropriate reaction. Other people's actions, opinions, and beliefs often cause irritation and anger, which directly affects your ability to communicate with others effectively. Anger makes you do irrational or unreasonable things. When you behave irrationally or unreasonably, others around you start to feel angry or resentful and threatened, thus creating a barrier in your effective communication. Anger not only affects you mentally but also has serious and detrimental effects on your physical health too. It increases adrenaline production, blood pressure, and heart rate. These factors can be harmful to your health in the long run.

## How to Recognize Anger?

Aggression and anger are two different things. Aggression is a type of behavior, while anger is a type of emotion. An angry person is not necessarily aggressive and vice versa. People often get aggressive when they feel threatened or afraid. People have different ways to let out their anger. Some get aggressive, some get sarcastic, and some become ignorant too. There are various emotional and physical signs by which you can recognize anger.

*Emotional Signs*

- A strong desire or feeling to lash out physically or verbally
- Anxiety
- Feeling resentful or guilty
- Feeling depressed or sad
- Feeling irritated
- A feeling to escape a situation

*Physical signs*

- Heightened cravings for comfort food, drugs, alcohol, sugar, tobacco, and so on
- Talking louder
- Loss of sense of humor
- Getting rude
- Pacing
- Difficulty to sit still
- Shaking or trembling hands and lips
- Sweaty palms
- Increase in heart rate
- Breathlessness or shallow breathing
- Grinding teeth or clenched jaw
- Clenched fists or a tight clasp of one hand with the other
- Rubbing the face frequently

## Types of Anger

There are various types of anger expression. Let us discuss some of them.

- **Assertive Anger** – This anger expression is of constructive type.

People having this type of anger expression are likely to use feelings of rage or frustration to fuel a positive change. These people don't resort to physical outbursts and verbal insults. They don't internalize anger or avoid confrontation. They are likely to act in ways that will help them meet their wants and needs and create change. They make sure not to cause any destruction or distress. When you express your anger assertively, it helps you to address your wants and needs in a very straightforward way, without defying other people's boundaries.

Assertive anger serves as a powerful motivator. Use it to achieve our life goals, address injustice, and overcome fears.

- **Behavioral Anger** – People having behavioral anger expression are likely to react physically. This expression of anger is physical, mainly aggressive, and sometimes even violent. This type of behavior has an intention to hurt someone who doesn't want it. These people are likely to throw or break things or attack or physically intimidate someone. When you express your anger using behavioral aggression, it can have negative interpersonal and legal consequences. This highly impulsive and unpredictable behavior diminishes your ability to form respectful and trusting relationships.

You should keep in mind that anger never generates violence or aggression automatically. Sit back and think about the real cause that made you choose aggression when you felt angry. When you start feeling angry, try removing yourself from that particular situation and practice self-talk to ground yourself at that time. You may regain control over your emotions in this way. You can even practice deep breathing to calm yourself down physically and reconsider the entire situation and think about the other different ways of reacting to this situation.

- **Chronic Anger** – People having chronic anger expression have a continuous feeling of resentment, frustration, and anger towards other people or even, sometimes, towards themselves. This ongoing sense of perpetual irritation and nagging can have adverse effects on their mental and physical wellbeing.

Spend some time and figure out the root cause of your anger. Once you find the source, you may find it easier to solve the conflict or to forgive others and yourself for whatever happened in the past. Forgiveness is empowering, and so it will help you to overcome your frustration and hurt. You can also learn to assertively express your emotions. This may be helpful, as well.

- **Judgmental Anger –** This type of anger expression is indignant, i.e., people who have judgmental anger expression react to situations that are perceived to be unfair or unjust. This anger expression is backed by a core belief of either superiority or inferiority. These people often tend to invalidate the difference of opinions with others.

Circumstances and situations are not always what they appear to be on the outside. Try to look at the bigger picture and don't be too fast to analyze a situation. Challenge your deep-rooted beliefs and assumptions and try to open up to the perspectives of other people. You may disagree at some points, but you may also get some insight into other people's perspectives and get a new angle of thinking and looking at things. It may be helpful for you to understand the situation when you try to understand it from others' perspectives as well.

- **Overwhelmed Anger –** This is an uncontrolled type of anger expression. It occurs when you feel that the water has risen above your head. When people feel that the situation is no longer in their hands, they show this kind of anger expression, which results in feelings of frustration and hopelessness. When people go through unexpected events in their lives, or when they take too much responsibility, it overthrows their natural stress-coping ability. This emotion is more like an alert that your patience level is about to break or things are about to get out of hands.

If you are experiencing this form of anger expression, you need to reach out to others and seek help. Share with your colleagues, friends, and family that you are feeling overwhelmed and that you need their help. Be vocal about what you need from them to feel secure and good. You can even make yourself busy with work. When you are occupied with work, your stress will alleviate, and thus you will regain behavioral and emotional control.

- **Passive-aggressive Anger** – This type of anger expression is avoidant. People having this particular type of anger expression evade all kinds of confrontation. They repress or deny any feelings of fury or frustration they are experiencing. Passive-aggressive anger is verbally expressed as veiled mockery, pointed silence, or sarcasm. It may also be physically expressed in behavior like delay in work, etc. People who express their anger in a passive way are not even aware that their actions are getting perceived as aggressiveness. This can have dreadful professional and personal outcomes.

Learn assertive communication and overcome the fear of confrontation.

- **Retaliatory Anger** – This type of anger expression is somewhat an involuntary response to being attacked or confronted by some other person. This type of anger expression is very common. It is motivated by revenge against something that is perceived as wrong. Vindictive anger can also be purposeful and deliberate. The aim is to intimidate people by exercising control over an outcome or a situation. This may end up escalating tensions.

Taking impulsive actions only worsens the situation. The only way to overcome it is to take some time and think before doing something.

- **Self-abusive Anger** – This type of anger expression is shame-based. If people feel ashamed, humiliated, unworthy, or hopeless, they may end up internalizing these feelings. They tend to vent their anger via disordered eating, substance use, self-harm, or negative self-talk. These people tend to lash out at others around them to mask their insecurities and low self-esteem.

  Learn cognitive reframing techniques and transform the distorted and self-defeating thoughts that you have been feeling. Meditation also helps to prevent you from engaging in self-harming activities.

- **Verbal Anger** – This type of anger expression is not as dangerous as behavioral anger expression, although it can deeply hurt the target's feelings due to the psychological and emotional abuse. It has violence and aggression and a motive to release it all by harming someone else. Verbal abuse is characterized by criticism or intense blaming, sarcasm, ridicule, threats, and furious shouting. People tend to feel regretful, apologetic, and ashamed after they have lashed out at someone.

  Think before you speak. The only way to cope with this type of anger is to prevent yourself from lashing out immediately and impulsively.

- **Volatile Anger** – People exhibiting volatile anger expression tend to get offended very quickly at both small and big issues. Once they vent their anger out, they are likely to calm down fast. This expression of anger may be destructive because people around you will tend to walk on eggshells to avoid triggering your rage. Volatile anger has adverse effects on your capacity to maintain long-term relationships. If not checked, volatile anger can lead to violent outbursts eventually.

Identify the symptoms and signs and then try relaxation techniques to prevent anger escalation.

## Signs That You Have Anger Management Issues

Are you unsure whether your anger levels are normal or not? If not, then check these signs and find it out yourself.

- **You are Passive-aggressive** – Passive-aggressiveness may look different than normal anger, but it is surely something serious. It is not violent or loud. Some people don't even understand that they are angry while experiencing passive-aggressiveness. When you are experiencing passive anger, your emotions may come out as meanness, apathy, or sarcasm. You may engage in self-harm and self-defeating behaviors like performing poorly in social or professional institutions, alienating family and friends, etc. People may think that you are doing these things intentionally, even when you may not even have any explanations for your actions.

- **You get Aggressive** – Every person feels angry, but not everyone fumes with rage. If you tend to verbally abuse, scream, or punch walls, then you certainly have anger management issues. Aggressive anger often gets displayed as retaliatory or volatile anger, and it can have physical damages to other people and properties. This form of anger can be dealt with by managing the anger symptoms and recognizing the factors that trigger the anger.

- **You Tend to Blame Others** – When you constantly blame others, it becomes easy to get angry. When state others responsible for your misery, it is very normal to get annoyed. Anger is not necessarily about what happened to you; rather, it is more about how you take and interpret things that happened to you. If you tend to blame others whenever something goes wrong, then you are surely having anger management issues.

- **You get Angry Frequently** – If you never find yourself chilled, then it is a problem. If you are always angry, then it is going to affect you both physically and mentally. It can have detrimental effects on your health, reputation, social life, jobs, relationships, etc. Think about yourself and the people around you and take the necessary actions to deal with your anger management issues.

- **You get Severely Angry at Petty Issues** – It is normal for people to feel angry, but it is nowhere near normal to get angry over small issues. This type of anger issue can make you injure or threaten others or even damage properties. It should be checked as early as possible to keep it manageable.

- **Your Anger is Long Lasting** – Sudden outbursts of anger are not good. Similarly, an everlasting rage is also not good. If it lasts too long, it can be a sign of a serious problem. If your anger is very frequent, intense, and long-lasting, you better get professional help, because otherwise it can be severely dangerous for you and the people around you.

# 2.
# Common Questions About Anger

One of the most common problems that people face these days is that of anger management issues because the times we live in are extremely stressful and full of testing situations cropping up. No matter how much we try, dealing with everything, that too, while keeping a cool mind, might not be an easy thing all the time. Thus, the majority of the people these days face anger management issues. For some, it might be something minor that they can deal with easily, but for others, this can be a huge problematic factor for which they need to take immediate action. Thus, in this article, we will talk about some of the very pertinent questions that generally crop up in people's minds regarding anger.

## Is There Only One Type of Anger?

A general misunderstanding about anger is that it can only bring problems and destruction. But that is the wrong idea. Anger can be both constructive and destructive. We can further break these up into finer categories, but first, let us talk about the constructive side of anger.

**Constructive anger** – Constructive anger has the capability to bring a healing opportunity to negative emotion. Though it might sound oxymoronic and can be quite challenging, yet a person can indeed use negative feelings in an optimistic way that might help him to heal, recover from a bad phase and move on towards something bright.

Anger can be triggered when a person does not contend with a given situation and is forced to speak up. Now objectively speaking, standing up for oneself can be a very good thing when the question comes up of boosting one's self-confidence. Instead of getting into an unwanted heated argument, a person can very well channelize this anger into a sensible discussion that will benefit everyone. With such an attitude, relationships, too, will improve over time with clearer communication between people. Constructive anger actually helps a person to become more understanding, creative, mindful, and conscious of his surroundings.

There can be various situations where no person but some external event can trigger anger. The trick lies as to how one can use that energy arising out of that anger to learn something new or to change the unfortunate situation into one of acceptance and resolution.

**Destructive anger** – Destructive anger is the one that we are unfortunately more familiar with than not. It can pass through different stages of varying destructive potential. The first is that of **Passive aggression**. In this case, the concerned person might derive certain sadistic pleasure out of purposefully doing something to disturb the other person to make them uncomfortable.

The next step can be that of **Sarcasm**, where the concerned person doesn't bother to hide his dislike about the other person and deliberately delivers derogatory remarks about him in order to taunt and hurt him personally.

The third step is that of **Silent treatment**, where the concerned person completely withdraws himself from doing any communication with the other person and choose to keep shut even if enquired about the same. This can greatly increase the miscommunication and intensify the problem.

Next comes **Hostility**, where the person can show his arrogance and annoyance openly. He doesn't hesitate to openly show signs of frustration and is also openly aggressive in his mode of speaking while having a conversation with the other person.

The last step is when the concerned person is openly **Aggressive** in his speech and actions both. It is in this stage that verbal fights might get dragged on to actual action with the associated people bad-mouthing one another. Serious damage to people and property might also occur as this might very well lead people to lose control.

## When it Comes to Anger, What to Believe and What Not to?

Like everything else, the issue of anger also has many false connotations attached to it that need to be get ridden of. There are certain myths about anger management issues that should not be trusted.

- The first thing that needs to be cleared is that *aggression* and *anger* are not the same. They are actually two very different modes of reaction to a given situation. On one side, it is true that a person becomes aggressive when he is extremely angry. But equating the two is wrong because anger when under control, doesn't bring destruction on its own. Thus, anger and aggression can only be brought together when the person loses control. Not otherwise.

- It is extremely important to realize that *ignoring* your anger can *never* be a way to deal with it. If a person thinks that ignoring the situation is the easy way out, well, it is not. Instead of providing a solution, ignoring the anger issue will only let it get bottled up. It can eventually lead to a situation where all these boxed up emotions burst out one day, bringing distress to everyone concerned.

- Some have this wrong notion that anger is just a *negative emotion*. This is completely false. Anger has many positive aspects to it as well, which, if taken into account, can bring many positive changes. Even history tells us that all major changes had taken place in the society as some people were angry with it and felt that it needed to be changed.

- One of the biggest myths regarding anger is that *anger management is not needed and is not efficient*. That is completely false. For those people who deal with anger management issues, getting a proper idea regarding one's situation and then taking effective steps to keep it under control is one of the most practical things to do. Not only is anger management needed, but it is also extremely effective.

- *Venting out one's anger is the best way to deal with it*. Well, this is not true at all. Though this is one way, this mostly has negative repercussions if a person can't keep his emotions under control. So instead of venting out one's anger, there are many alternative ways in which anger can be dealt with where none of the concerned people gets hurts physically or verbally.

## Does Anger Affect Everyone in the Same Way?

It is true that some people tend to get angrier than others. At the same time, two different people might react to a certain situation in two very different ways, even if they are similarly affected by it and are both angry. So why does that happen? That happens because how much a person is prone to anger is depended on many factors like his thoughts, physical activities he indulges in, and also his psychological framework. Some people are very sensitive when it comes to responding to stimuli. These people tend to get overboard with their feelings very easily. A slight touch or smell or noise is enough to hamper their balance, and they tend to react negatively. While the other category won't really mind these issues, and even if they are slightly uncomfortable, they will choose to ignore it rather than get angry and create a scene.

There might be a few other factors here that play a very important role in how tolerant people are when it comes to anger. Habits play a major role in people's lives. At the same time, how a child has been brought up is to be taken into consideration when measuring his anger issues. Kids who have grown up in an abusive or careless environment are more prone to have trouble managing their anger. Plus, those individuals who are into gaming and genuinely enjoy violent games are more prone to give in to violent behaviors than others. The same goes for people who enjoy violent movies or music that falls under such a category.

## How Can I Differentiate Between Healthy and Unhealthy Anger?

As mentioned earlier in the article, anger can be broadly classified between constructive anger, which we can even call healthy anger, and destructive anger, which we can be termed as unhealthy anger. It depends on how the concerned person is reacting to that present situation and what steps he is taking to get a remedy. The person might choose the energy that anger is creating in him to take a positive step and change things for the better. The person might also decide to become violent and worsen the situation further. Whether one can keep the anger within range to a feeling of annoyance or be filled with rage is also dependent on many factors.

What is important to keep in mind here is to take notice as to what are the things that are causing this anger. Anger can be triggered when a person is denied what he wants or what he feels that he deserves. This might lead to frustration. Now, if this want is legitimate, then getting angry is justified, as that arises out of the need to be treated respectfully. But if this anger is caused just because certain things didn't turn out the way a person wanted, irrespective of it being justified or not, then that is a problem.

But this might be a problem as it can be difficult to differentiate between the two as the lines between the two can get really blurry. Look for certain signs if you are confused. See whether this anger is making you deny your own feelings and whether you are opting for violence as a defense mechanism. That definitely falls under unhealthy anger. If, on the other hand, you are able to able to compartmentalize your feelings and to steer them towards taking constructive steps in your life, then that anger is definitely healthy.

## Does Our Health Suffer Due to Anger?

This is a very common question that is asked by a majority of people who deal with anger management issues. Anger does many things to our bodies. Due to a sudden increase in the stress hormone level in our body released by the adrenal glands, the blood that was supposed to flow towards our brain gets directed to our muscles, which gives rise to excitement, fear, and anxiety. As a result, a person might face a peak in his concentration level and get inertia to buckle up and get things done. But in some extreme cases, the vital signs of the body can get affected due to a wild flow of hormones bringing grave consequences. Hence, there comes a high risk of diseases like hypertension, gastric ulcers, heart attacks, strokes, or panic attacks.

## When Does Anger Management Become Necessary?

Anger management is one of the essential requirements when it comes to leading a balanced life. Not only do people who suffer from anger issues should practice it, but these practices are beneficial or everyone. Thus, anger management is indeed essential. But it is true that some people will need it more urgently than others.

If you feel that you are resorting to negative means to deal with your anger or trying to avoid the real issue by hiding behind baseless aggression, anger management skills need to be practiced. You might not be a violent person necessarily, but you might grow that tendency by finding yourself unable to keep your emotions in check. This might be a problem in the long run. In such cases, anger management skills are needed as such tendencies will drive your near ones away, which might cause a problem in your professional front.

## Should Dealing With Anger Between Family and Strangers Be Different?

A certain thing that we need to keep in mind is that when it comes to family members, we get many chances to communicate with them, and hence both the chances of getting angry with them and making up for it increases. So, if a certain family issue or member is making you angry, try communicating with that person at the earliest as otherwise, it might give rise to uncomfortable situations. But when it comes to strangers whom we might not meet again, that one instant of rudeness can leave a negative impression forever. Such situations are better to be avoided.

These are some of the most commonly asked questions regarding anger, which hopefully we have provided satisfactory answers for.

# 3.
# What Triggers Your Anger?

There can be various reasons for a person's anger. It may be a response to threats, a way to protect the loss of some possessions, protect family members or territory, etc. The reasons behind your anger may sometimes be irrational and sometimes rational, too (if the reasons are mostly irrational, it means that you have anger management issues). The causes of anger vary from person to person. Anger is not about the situations you face, but the way you interpret that situation and react to it. This is why triggering elements of anger varies hugely from person to person. A thing that triggers your anger may be completely fine with someone else and vice versa. So, if your interpretation of some situation is different than those of others, it doesn't mean that you are wrong. If you are angry at something which others don't find angry at all, it doesn't necessarily mean that your anger is not justified. Everyone is unique, and their perceptions vary hugely. Interpreting a particular situation depends greatly on a few factors.

Let us discuss them.

- **Current Circumstances** – If a lot of things are going on in your life right now, then you are likely to feel angry at petty issues. You can even get angry unreasonably. If in a particular situation, which triggers your anger, you fail to vent out your anger, then you may find yourself venting out anger at other situations meaninglessly. If you have recently lost someone dear to you, you will find it very difficult to cope with all the things happening around you, leading to depression, irritation, and sometimes anger.

- **Past Experiences** – If you have had past experiences that were bitter, for example, bullying, trauma, or abuse, and if you were unable to vent your anger at that time, then it is possible that you may still struggle to cope with those feelings now. Because of your bitter experiences, you may find situations that will seem challenging and difficult to cope with. Your present frustration and anger are not necessarily based on something in the present. Past experiences play a vital role. Once you become aware of this, it will be a lot easier for you to handle these challenging situations tactfully.

- **Childhood Experiences and Upbringing** – The way you cope with your anger issues are directly influenced by your upbringing. Many people have been told certain things about anger as a child, and that affects their ability to handle anger even when they are grownups.

    While growing up, you may have been thinking that it is okay to act out violently or aggressively if you are angry. This may be the reason that you did not learn how to manage your anger. As a result, you have violent outbursts whenever something doesn't go your way.

    You may have been thinking that it is not okay to complain. You may have been receiving punishments in your childhood to express anger. As a result, you have developed a habit of suppressing your anger. This makes it a long-term issue. And so, you tend to have violent outbursts frequently because you don't know how to release your anger in a healthy way. It may even be self-destructive.

- You may have seen your parents or other grownups in their angriest moments when they reacted violently. This may have created a sense of terror within you as a child. You may have been thinking of anger as something destructive, violent, and scary. Thus, you are afraid of your own anger and don't want to express it because of the fear of the consequences. As a result, you may have sudden violent outbursts in the most inappropriate and unexpected situations, thus making things worse for you.

## Importance of Knowing Your Anger Triggers

- It is very important to know your own anger triggers. Instead of trying to manage the situation after having an angry outburst, try to prevent it from happening in the first place. In order to prevent it from happening, you need to, at first, know the factors contributing to your anger. Once you become aware of your anger triggers, it becomes very easy to circumvent your anger.

- Once you understand your anger triggers, you will be able to anticipate your anger episodes. Once you anticipate, you will be able to prevent that episode from happening and intentionally react in some other way for the time being. When you are well aware of your triggers, you will be able to choose how to react. You should be more observational about the factors that are going to trigger you, and you should take necessary measures to talk yourself into a much calmer and appropriate response instead of an aggressive one.

- The self-control that you maintain while understanding the things that are going on in your brain helps you to be in charge of your own reactions while angry. As a result, your emotions and thoughts remain in your cortex so that you stay rational and strategic instead of irrational and impulsive.

Although factors that trigger your anger vary from person to person, let us discuss some of the most common triggers to anger.

- Sadness or grief may trigger anger. Examples include the loss of a loved one, family member, or a friend that may serve as a trigger to your anger.

- If you are mentally or physically unwell, then it can be your trigger. People who are seriously ill or are in pain tend to stay frustrated and angry.

- If something wrong is done to you or to someone you care about, it can trigger your anger. Examples include mistreatment, sexual offenses, violence, theft, etc.

- Taking alcohol and drugs may trigger your anger. Even leaving them can be frustrating and trigger anger.

- Disappointment and failure may also trigger anger.

- Stress is a very common factor that triggers anger. It can be your work stress or something in your personal life, which can make you stay irritated most of the time.

- Financial problems may also trigger your anger.

- If you are sexually frustrated, then it can be a trigger to your anger.

- Injustice or something which is considered to be wrongdoing may often trigger anger. Embarrassment, humiliation, getting bullied, etc. are a few examples.

- Hunger can also be a reason for your anger. When you are hungry, then everything except mood makes you angry.

- Tiredness can be a major trigger to your anger. Short-tempered people tend to get very irritated when they are tired.

- Poor interpersonal skills and rudeness also serve as triggers to your anger.

## The Relationship between Anger and Trauma

A very common response to trauma is anger. High ager levels are directly related to a person's natural survival instinct. When you face extreme threats, you tend to behave with anger. Anger makes that person shift his focus from the ongoing trauma, thus making him survive through it. When something seems unfair to you, or you feel victimized by a certain situation, anger comes as a common response. Studies have shown that when you get betrayed by others, you tend to get angry. Angry responses are seen mostly in situations that involve violence or exploitation. In the case of childhood abuse, the shock and trauma of those events affect the way the survivor learns to take charge of his or her emotions. Trauma may lead to frequent violent outbursts of extreme emotions like rage and anger.

Even though we are going to study the anger management strategies in detail in the latter part of this book, here are some things that you can do –

- It is really difficult to keep control over yourself when you are fuming with rage; still, it is not entirely impossible. It is tough to talk yourself down from that situation. It is better to avoid such a situation in the first place. Learn to take hints and understand just when exactly you are just starting to get angry. Once you recognize the signs, take a step back, and try different relaxation techniques to prevent the escalation of your irritation and anger.

- Stop dwelling in the past. Some people have a habit of digging skeletons, which is very harmful in this case. There is no use in going on and on over some incident that has already occurred and has been sorted out. Try to let things go and move on. One effective way to do this is by focusing on the positive side of each and every person in a situation.

- You should change your ways of thinking in order to keep a check on your anger. When you are angry, things seem more frustrating than they actually are. Use cognitive restructuring as a way to replace negative and unhelpful thoughts in your brain with positive and reasonable ones. Instead of thinking that it is the end of the world, you should start practicing to think of the situation as tough but not the worst.

- You should not use words such as "always" or "never" while talking about others or yourself. Statements involving these words tend to give you a feeling that your anger is justified, thus making it harder for you to cope with the situation. This may also lead to the alienation of people who would have otherwise worked with you or stayed by your side.

- Try to use logic. Even when your anger is justified, it takes no time to make you irrational. Always remember that this world is not your enemy. There is always a way to fight every crisis, and you will be able to do it too if you want to. Whenever you start feeling angry, remind yourself this so that you feel more positive, rather than feeling negative all the time.

- Convert your expectations into desires. People who are angry often start demanding things because of their will to do things their way. Instead of demands, try to make requests. Even if things don't turn out the way you planned them to be, don't let your disappointment or sadness turn into agitation or anger. Take things lightly in a positive way.

- Try to relax. Certain relaxing techniques are very helpful in situations like these. You can try muscle relaxation. You can tense your muscles and then slowly relax them one at a time. This will help you to get a calmer mind. You can even try imagining relaxing and soothing things. This will help your brain to calm itself down. You can even try focused breathing. When you are angry, you tend to do shallow breathing. Try to practice well-controlled breathing. In this way, you will be able to bring yourself back to a calmer state.

- Improve your communication skills. Be vocal about what are your likes and dislikes. In this way, you will be able to prevent many such unwanted situations. If you are vocal about your likes and dislikes, you are less likely to get involved in a situation that you dislike. This is because people around you are already aware of that and so they will make sure that you don't have to face such situations. In case you have already found yourself in such a situation, make sure that you talk it out instead of reacting violently. Talk about how that made you upset and what can be done to make it better. In this way, you will be able to save yourself from acting out violently.

- Try physical exercise. If you exercise regularly, it may help you to get over your anger. Exercising regularly liberates both your mind and body. You may even try meditation. Meditation relaxes your mind and plays a vital role in controlling your emotions. Meditate on a regular basis, and only then will you be able to control your emotions.

The world is a beautiful place, and we should not waste time feeling angry or frustrated. It only makes things worse. It is better to handle things in a calmer way instead of acting out; otherwise, it gets really difficult for you and the people around you. You may unknowingly hurt others due to this behavior. If you still can't control your anger, try seeking medical help.

# 4.
# In What Ways Is Anger a Problem?

In humans, a natural instinctive response to threats can be anger. Though certain kinds of anger might be necessary as that becomes a coping mechanism for our survival, yet anger, in most cases, can become a problem if you fail to keep it under control. The moment your anger goes out of your control, it might lead you to give in to your vulnerabilities, making you do or say things that you will regret later. Uncontrolled anger, in most cases, leads to physical and emotional illness, harming the person concerned and also having a harmful impact on others if they are unfortunate enough to find themselves a victim in such a situation as violence is a common by-product of uncontrolled rage.

## When Can Anger Cause Real Trouble?

Anger can start creating trouble if it starts coming in the way of other daily works that a person is doing, hampering the concerned person and others around. With prolonged anger, a person might become aggressive, unfeeling, unresponsive, and even hurtful. Having trouble controlling this anger may have serious consequences. The person might start keeping to himself and declining social interactions. In some other cases, a person might also feel the need to harm oneself and others in that state of anger induced frenzy. This will have a negative impact on one's social as well as personal life. This will also lead to a feeling of serious regret on the part of the concerned person, which is further bad for mental and physical health.

## Effects That Anger Can Have On the Health of a Person

Anger affects different parts of the body. While those who lash out violently, anger has different repercussions on the concerned person and others around; for those who tend to hold in their anger, it has different physical and psychological impacts that might lead to various problems.

### Physical Effects

Our body has different ways of dealing with various negative situations. Likewise, when it comes to managing stress, anger is one of the coping mechanisms our body develops. But what happens, as a result, is that there is an increase in heartbeat and also high blood pressure. Though the body is able to deal with the normal level of stress that one has to face every day, yet when it becomes too much to handle, the internalizing effects of anger on a person's health is harmful as it might destabilize the internal balance of certain hormones. Extreme cases might also lead to the body falling victim to various diseases leading to an early death.

Medical research has shown that the stress response of anger can lead to a patient developing

- Elevated blood pressure (a condition in which the force of the blood against the artery walls is too high and might lead to a stroke),

- Increased heart rate (a condition where the heart rate is above a hundred beats per hour,

- A kind of a heart rhythm disorder that might lead to heart failure),

- Tensing of muscles (with a high amount of stress level, the muscles tend to tense up at the same time only to release this tension when the moment of stress passes),

- Migraine is a result of such muscle tensing,

- Hiatal hernia (a condition where a part of the stomach pushes up through diaphragm muscle causing heartburn and abdominal discomfort),

- Glaucoma (an eye condition that can cause blindness as the nerve connecting the eye to the brain gets damaged),

- Urticaria ( a skin condition where rashes come up on the skin resulting from medicinal effect, food or stress, and anger),

- Asthma (a person's airways get inflamed, producing extra mucus, making it difficult to breathe; extreme conditions can be life-threatening as well),

- Ulcer (a sore that develops on the lining of the oesophagus, small intestine, or stomach),

- Lower back pain (a very painful condition affecting the lower regions of the spine),

- Insomnia (a condition where the affected person might suffer from sleeplessness),

- Psoriasis (it is an immune system problem triggered due to stress and anger, cold or infections where the skin cells build up and form scales, becoming itchy and extremely dry),

- High levels of stress hormones that are linked with feelings of anger can affect the lungs a lot by inflaming the airways, and overall the life expectancy can get reduced by a great level.

## Psychological Effects

The mental health of a person can be hugely affected by a condition of constant anger and stress. A person might develop a series of different psychological issues that might make conducting oneself quite problematic. Issues like anxiety disorders or loneliness, or depression are very common signs that occur in people dealing with anger issues. People who have clinical depression tend to shut their emotions by suppressing them in order to cope up with their life. This might lead them to get violent suddenly, and a sudden angry outburst is very common. This suppressed anger might also trigger self- harm on the part of this concerned person, and harming those near him might also become a possibility. Eating disorders and sleeping disorders are also very common. Different kinds of phobias and OCD, also known as Obsessive-compulsive disorder, can also be located among people dealing with anger issues. As a result, the effects of anger can have a deep-rooted impact on a person's professional and public life, making it difficult to function efficiently.

The stress hormones present in our body are cortisol, adrenaline, and noradrenaline. What anger does is increase the level of cortisol, which in turn causes a loss of neurons in the PCF, that is, the prefrontal cortex. This condition stops a person from making proper judgments and making decisions. An elevated cortisol level in the brain will also kill the neurons present in the hippocampus and will also disrupt the formation of new neurons. As a result, the short- term memory is weakened.

Anger prevents forming new memories, and that is the reason a person might find it difficult to remember what he said during an argument.

Anger can also lead to an attitude of self- victimization as the concerned person won't really get what is wrong on his part as getting angry and reacting in the way he does is fully justified to him. That person will also fail to realize what a bad precedent he is setting up for others and how negatively it is hampering the lives of those around him. Hence, the concerned person might fail to realize why he is getting distanced from others or being avoided by those near him. As a result, the concerned person might feel that this a conscious decision on the other person's part, making him feel like a victim, which in turn is a result of his own misdoings.

## Effects That Anger Can Have On Intimate Relationships

Not only does anger affect the concerned person, but it also has a mild to severe impact on the personal relationships that the person is having. Angry exchanges between the couple might lead to a communication gap. Problems might range from mild discomforts to explosive verbal or physical exchanges that might cumulate to serious damage over time.

Anger makes a person defensive of his vulnerabilities and underlying emotions. As the person on the other side of the miscommunication fails to understand the true feelings, this might also lead that person to act defensively to that anger. This ultimately results in two upset people who are misreading the underlying reasons for each other's actions.

A person might develop various negative traits due to the underlying anger issues that will invariably hamper the relationship. Things like snapping at each other for any simple thing that doesn't match the frequency or nitpicking at each other's habits and choices might accumulate as resentments, which might lead to an eruptive behavior on one or both the parts one day. Hurtful accusations and explosive threats hamper the trust in a relationship.

Anger and stress make a person increasingly resentful with time if one partner is made to be the victim of the other's hateful behavior all the time. A patronizing behavior on the partner's part silences the other, which lets the relationship lose its strength. Quite naturally, the attitude of the couple becomes cold towards each other, with one partner resorting to an attitude of withdrawal in order to avoid further problems. It can also happen that the other partner might choose to never say anything or voice out their true feelings, silently accepting everything. This will also lead to the couple losing trust in each other as there remains no space for open communication anymore.

One of the easiest ways that people choose to deal with such abusive relationships is alcohol and drugs. This might also lead to the couple seeking comfort outside the relationship. These may seem to be the temporary easy answer yet is never the actual solution. When angry, a person might also seek revenge on the other partner, which might be the most destructive in a relationship. Anger makes a person want to vanquish the other. Thus, a person might stoop down to using derogatory statements about the other person. Character assassination is also very common. Rage can make a person lose out on basic manners as a result of which one might very easily attack the other person based on their most vulnerable traits, threatening to leave them. The angry predating partner feels a constant need to win all the time, which urges them to continue this kind of behavior.

It is thus understandable how much a personal relationship might get hampered due to anger issues on the part of one or both the partners.

## Effects That Anger Can Have On Your Workplace

Our professional lives take up a large chunk of our day to day activities. No matter what work we invest ourselves in, be it during our educative years, where we move from one institution to another, or after we take up jobs, our workplaces always hold a special place in our lives. It thus becomes extremely important to maintain a proper code of conduct in all such places. A will to learn, a positive attitude towards team play, an understanding outlook towards fellow colleagues, the ability to retain one's calm under pressure, a never- be-defeated attitude towards failure, a willingness to accept one's faults and starting afresh without keeping any grudges are some qualities that every professional front expects out of its employees. No matter what field we choose to work in, these qualities are extremely important for any person to grow and learn. If taken notice, it is these very things that a person having anger management issues finds himself lacking in because all of these needs a certain amount of patience and self- control that this concerned person might not have.

Frustration due to work, unfair treatment from the boss or seniors, interpersonal conflicts, excessive workload, late office hours are all very common scenarios that might occur in every person's life. These very easily induce anger and irritation. Problems might occur if someone has difficulties in keeping this anger in check. It is useless to expect an ideal work environment as that rarely exists. So, in this case, these unfavorable situations will invariably lead the person to react in a negative way. It might be a trigger to explosive outbursts, violent actions, threats, and shouts and, in extreme cases, quitting one's job. Even if the person is able to keep one's job, such behavior will be the cause of a very bad reputation and might even lead to an eventual termination from the job. Your colleagues will start ignoring you, and as a result, there will be little to no progress in one's workplace.

## Effects That Anger Can Have On An Unborn Child of a Pregnant Women

It is true that the months of pregnancy are usually very tough for any given woman as the body and the mind of the mother go through various changes, and as a result, a woman might not always be in the best of her spirits. However, it should be known that frequent stress and anger can have serious ill effects on the health of both the mother and the unborn child. For example, anger might lead to an increase in the mother's blood pressure, and subsequently, the heart rate will also increase, both of which are very bad for the unborn child. Hormones like epinephrine and adrenaline may shoot up, which will constrict the blood vessels of the mother. What happens as a result is that the blood supply and the oxygen supply of the fetus get reduced to a great extent and might even be fatal for the child.

Prolonged anger and stress have a negative impact on the mother even during the time of pregnancy as the baby might have very low birth weight and there might be a certain unfavorable impact on the baby's temperament; that is, after birth, the baby might be prone to depression and other such psychological issues. In certain extreme cases, the baby might also have to be delivered prematurely. There are high chances of the baby being hyperactive as well.

## Effects That Anger Can Have on Friendships

A person might fail to realize this, but the effects of anger and its subsequent behavior might be a cause of great distress for others around that person, especially if that person is our friend. For those near us, we might choose not to point out our mistakes all the time or might choose to ignore it more often than not in the hope of not hurting us or elevating the anger by giving more importance to the situation at hand. What it does is create miscommunication and a slow but deep distance between the concerned friends. A friend might understand us more to not jump to conclusions at our slightest change in behavior. But if a person has anger management issues and the other person becomes a constant victim of that toxic behavior, then with time, either the friend will stop communicating all together or will accept everything in the hope of things getting better someday, which might not happen at all. In both the scenarios, the friendship gets hampered, bringing a very evident and sad bridge between the two. In any relationship, respecting the other person is a necessity, which people with anger management issues tend to forget or ignore.

In conclusion, anger is really a huge problem that might have serious consequences if ignored or developed over time, which will make the personal and public life of the concerned person extremely difficult and problematic. It has the ability to cause havoc if not taken care of immediately. Along with having a severe physical illness, it will also make the concerned person succumb to serious psychological ailments that might require prolonged treatment for cure. It is thus, better to deal with anger management issues at the earliest.

# 5.
# Control Anger Before It Controls You

Anger is a very common emotion that every single one of us experiences on a regular basis in our lives. However, anger is also an emotion that has the potentials to cause some amount of ugliness and discomfort in both our lives and the lives of people around us; therefore, it is important to know and learn how to keep anger and the outbursts caused by it under check. Listed below are some tips and tricks which you can utilize in your daily life in order to keep your anger in check:

## Take a Time Out

Taking a time out is one of the most effective things to do if you are in the middle of a heated argument with someone. Simply take a time out and tell them that you need a break from the argument at hand and will come back to it later. This is respectful of both your and the other person's private space, and with a time out, you can simply walk away. This might help you gain a fresh perspective on things and maybe deal with not just your anger but also the entire situation in a better and more mature way. But make sure that the time out, or break, is not a permanent thing! Set a boundary between the both of you, and also set a time and place where you will get back to the argument and finish it. Do not leave the discussion unattended for a very long time, as that might lead to either (or both) of you holding onto a grudge, which is perhaps a lot unhealthier.

## Think About Possible Triggers

Is there a specific topic of conversation or a particular incident from your past, which spoils your mood whenever it is brought up, regardless of the situation or context? If that is so, it is a possible trigger for your anger, and it is helpful to let people around you know that you are not comfortable with talking about that particular topic. If the topic is something you absolutely cannot avoid, then it might be helpful to inform people that you will bring it up when you feel comfortable talking about it, and they can have a discussion on it with you then.

## Try to Change Your Routine

Think hard about whether there are certain aspects of your daily routine, which automatically put you in a bad mood. It could be a part of your daily commute, it could be the service at the place you go for your mid-work coffee, or it could even be a good morning message from someone you'd rather not see in your notifications. If there are situations that just do not sit well with you and make you feel frustrated or angry, the best way to deal with them is to switch up your daily routine. Make small changes and spread them out over time so that you are not significantly altering your daily routine but are slowly getting rid of all the minor triggers which could pile on to a bad mood.

## Say It In Your Head First

When you are in the middle of an argument, a lot of things you say can be very hurtful. Many times, these are absolutely uncalled for and are not things you would say intentionally. In the heat of the moment, you can say some of such things, but what would happen is that they might cause long term damage and would hurt the person at the receiving end, perhaps beyond repair. So, in order to preserve friendships and relationships, what can work very well is to say what you want to say out loud once in your head first because once the words are out there, there is no taking them back. Saying it in your head will also help you put yourself in the other person's shoes and understand how those words would impact you if you were on the receiving end. Accordingly, you can then choose to either say or not say it or tweak a few things out in how you choose to respond. What also helps sometimes- especially if the argument is happening online, over text messages, or something similar- is to write down what you want to tell the other person in your Notes app or somewhere else private. After you are feeling a little more composed and the anger has subsided, you can go back and take a look at it and decide accordingly if that is an appropriate response to send across or not.

## Hear Other Perspectives Out

There is no easier way to put this, but a lot of times, we are very angry simply because we are way too caught up in the way we choose to see things. When someone else's world view does not align with ours, it might cause us to get a little uncomfortable and even angry at times because we cannot compel anyone else to see and understand things in the exact way that we do. However, it might help if we hear the other person out and get a sense of their perspective because, in all probabilities, they are equally frustrated with the fact that we do not see things the way they do. If both of you could patiently hear each other out and reach a middle ground with some sort of agreement to respect your differences while maintaining your original standpoint, a lot of conflict and anger could be easily kept aside.

## Talk It Out With a Third Person

Talking of different perspectives, another useful way to deal with anger is to talk things out with a third person, that is, someone who is completely unfamiliar with the argument and, therefore, is also completely neutral and unbiased if it might come to picking sides. Discussing the issue at hand with them and hearing their perspective can greatly influence you in terms of how you approach the conversation on your own. Also, the high chances are that if the fight is about something very trivial in the first place, a third person will call you out for making a huge deal out of something which is not very important, and then you can perhaps drop the argument altogether, which will go on to save everyone involved a lot of time and energy.

## Channel the Energy Somewhere Else

Anger and any outbursts related to anger comes with a gush of energy, which is often channelized in a negative way through shouting, picking a fight, etc. However, one of the things you can do is to take that energy and channel it somewhere else, preferably doing a positive or constructive activity. A lot of people actually clean their room or organize stuff when they are angry or frustrated because refocusing your attention to create a decluttered physical space can often help in decluttering your headspace as well. However, you do not necessarily have to clean. Pick an activity you have been setting aside for a long time, something that will require you to actively divert your attention and energy to finish it, and get onto it! Before you realize, you will probably be done with it (thanks to all the energy from your pent up anger), and you will also have taken enough time off from conflict for you to look back at it from a fresh perspective. Or even better, you might feel that the situation did not warrant an angry reaction from you to start with, and you would not need to go back.

## Focus On 'I' Statements

If you are angry and are in an ongoing argument, make sure to focus on using statements that begin with 'I' instead of statements that begin with 'You.' A prime example of this would be saying, "I am unable to understand what you are trying to convey" instead of "You are wrong and make no sense." While 'you' sentences tend to place blame on the other person and make it look like they are the one completely at fault in this situation, 'I' sentences bring you into the picture and acknowledge that you are falling short in one way or the other in dealing with the situation at hand. It also implies that you are already working on your side of the problem by identifying where you have gone wrong and are most likely also willing to fix your behavior so that the conflict can be resolved. 'I' based sentences, in other words, are just more actionable in nature and place the responsibility of your side of the argument on you, instead of passively blaming someone else and expecting them to do the combined work of two people to fix the situation. Even otherwise, saying things like "I need a break" instead of "You got to give me a break" puts your needs first in the exchange and implies that you are setting healthy boundaries, which actually works better in forming a healthy channel of communication, no matter what the nature of the conversation is.

## Maintain a Journal

Maintaining a journal is a really good idea, and it will help you process not just anger but a lot of other emotions as well, in a very healthy way. A journal is a handy solution if you want to vent things out. Keep it in mind that although venting it out to a friend is one way of dealing with things, everyone has their personal boundaries, and you must not overburden anybody else and exhaust them of their capacity to hear you out as well. Therefore, if you are feeling very consumed and really want to vent out, one of the foolproof ways to do it simply write it down- be it using the classic pen and paper method or on a Word document. Make sure to ensure that your journal- digital or physical- is a safe space for your thoughts, and take all precautions required to ensure that. It might mean keeping your laptop password protected or storing your journal in a place where nobody will access it without your consent. Having a steady journal can also help you to reflect upon past incidents and spot any pattern in your behavior and reactions over time, which will, in turn, help you identify problematic behavior and rectify it so that you are better in charge of how you feel and react to situations.

## Empathy Goes a Long Way

Empathy is one of the most important life skills, and training yourself consciously to be more empathetic can actually help you a lot, in different ways. Even when it comes to dealing with anger, empathy is perhaps the most useful skill you can equip yourself with. This would not just help you see things from someone else's point of view and fathom the sort of effect the argument is having on them; it would even help you out if a second party is not involved in the conflict at all. You must keep in mind that any emotional outburst you have would affect not just you but also multiple people around you- be it your support system, the people you live with, the people you work with, and many others. You being in a spoiled mood might have a lasting impact on them in different magnitudes, and nobody else should have to suffer in any way because of your emotional outbursts because most of them are not even related to you in that close a capacity. If you are empathetic enough, you will recognize the fact that you must cut everyone around you slack and not let your anger come in their way of doing things, which in turn will help you reflect upon how you deal with and control your anger. Practicing empathy regularly will really help you out, this way, in controlling negative emotions all throughout your life.

## Consider Possible Solutions

A lot of situations which make you angry most likely have a practical solution which can be worked out. This does not mean that the emotion you feel towards the situation is unwarranted or trivial, but it just means that your reaction could have been a very impulsive one, and once that stage has passed, it might help to take an analytical approach towards the conflict so that you can figure out whether it can be solved or not. If there are possible and realistic solutions, then it is highly suggested to try a few of them out- not just at that very moment, but also beforehand if you face a similar situation in the future, so that you can do away with the impulsive reaction then. It is also possible that the conflict that caused you to get angry in the first place might not have any possible solution at all, and if that is the case, then it is perhaps best to let things be and just get on with your life.

## Holding a Grudge Can Be Harmful

One of the ugliest things that can come out of anger is a long term grudge. Holding a grudge against someone can be extremely harmful because if you have a grudge, the chances are that you are going to be unfairly biased in any future interaction you would have with the person concerned. And also, in the longer run, you are most likely to forget a lot of details about what caused the grudge in the first place, and what will remain is the feeling of unease and dislike between the two of you, which can be conveniently done away with, because it does no good for either party involved. Talking things out sometimes after an argument is one of the best ways to ensure you are not holding any unresolved grudges against another person. Also, reversely, if you feel like you have moved past an argument you had with someone else, but they might have not, it is a good idea to have a heart to heart conversation with them. It might just have been that they were not very aware of your side of things and had been holding an unwarranted grudge against you all this time, without you realizing.

## Have a Go-To Mode of Relaxation

This is a good thing to figure out even if you are someone who is not prone to having angry outbursts. Trying out different modes of relaxation and finding one that works for you in any given situation is a huge plus point to keep your mind away from any sort of overwhelming emotions. For some people, this might be taking a walk; for others, it could be listening to a well-curated playlist on Spotify, and for someone else, it could just be to plug their devices off and take a nap. These strategies vary from people to people and are very subjective, so it is important that you try a few out and see what works the best for you. Here, it might not be very helpful to rely completely on what other people suggest (you can use them as a starting point, but do not settle on it) because obviously, just like triggers for anger are not the same for all people, how they can relax to take their mind off from that situation is also different.

## Compartmentalize Your Emotions

Well, to begin with, compartmentalization might not be a very healthy coping mechanism. However, it can work out very well sometimes when there are too many things on your plate, and you do not want to spend all your energy on conflict resolution. How you can compartmentalize your emotions during an anger outburst is to simply shift your focus to a different task at hand and tell yourself that the thing you are angry at does not matter for the moment, and you will go back to it perhaps after you have completed five other tasks, or maybe at the end of that day. In this way, this step is also a lot like taking a time out, except here, the deal you are making with is not another person, but yourself. So, when you are very angry, and you feel like a lot of your time is being consumed by a certain conflict, draw yourself up a quick to-do list (start with very basic and doable tasks) and stay focused on finishing them step by step.

## Seeking Help is Important

Everything said and done; we need to understand which anger-related outbursts are normal and which ones are not. If you are experiencing anger more frequently and more intensely than you earlier used to (or that people around you usually do), and if you feel like none of the strategies mentioned above is effectively helping you to keep your anger under check, then it might be time to seek professional help about your anger issues. Anger counseling is absolutely normal, and more people than you think seek it on a normal basis, so there is absolutely no need to get negatively influenced by any sort of stigma about seeking professional counseling if you feel like you could benefit from it. Seeking help is important, and what is even more important is being able to identify when things are serious enough for you to seek help. In such a situation, it might be useful to also take into consideration what other people, who are close to you, are saying because the chances are that they might be able to identify when you need professional help before you do. If there is a trusted friend or family member whom you fall back on usually during distressing times, and they express concern, then it might be a good time to consider how you can go about seeking help from there. You also need to keep in mind that although your loved ones are there to listen to you and give you advice, they cannot substitute the kind of help you would get from a trained counselor.

# 6.
# CBT for Anger Management

Anger is better known as a normal human emotion. In a maximum number of cases, anger has proven to be a sort of weakness, but a lot of people think that anger needs to be treated as a strength. In reality, a person who displays anger possesses less inner strength than the one who avoids displaying it. If you take the example of fire, then you will notice that besides hurting you, fire hurts or is harmful to other people as well. Similarly, if you show anger and fail to control it, then the spark of anger will burn you at first and then the others. Yes, it is true that anger is one of the most common outbursts of emotions present in almost all individuals.

It usually occurs when something happens against your expectations. It occurs when you expect someone to treat you fairly, but they don't. You expect your children to obey the desires of elders, but sometimes they fail to do so. Whenever a gap is created between reality and expectation, anger runs in for filling in that particular gap. Another usual cause of anger is when you get to notice imperfection around you, and you are incapable of accepting it. Anger is fine if you are able to press the 'delete' button as soon as you realize that your anger is rising. But, when a person is unable to control anger, then a huge number of problems arise in almost every single part of life: emotional, mental, physical, and others. Anger is not at all good, and thus it needs to be controlled or prevented, or managed.

It is very difficult to define uncontrolled anger. Individuals who experience uncontrolled anger fail to realize its long-term results, and that is actually a huge problem. Such consequences may include health-related problems such as high chances of intense heart disease, high blood pressure, and a lot more. It even has other ill effects like creating social conflict among friends, co-workers, family members, relatives, etc. If you or your closed ones suffer from uncontrolled anger, then you need not worry as various ways do exist for controlling or treating anger. Some of the means of controlling anger include yoga, regular meditation, taking deep breaths, therapies, etc. A lot of authentic research studies state the fact that therapies are highly effective for dealing with anger. One such well-known therapy is CBT or cognitive-behavioral therapy. A maximum number of researches that are done on the treatment of anger have a focus on CBT, which is one of the most common forms of psychotherapy or talk therapy.

Cognitive-behavioral therapy may assist you in managing the problems that you face because of anger by altering your thinking process or thoughts and behavior. Here you will get to know all about CBT and its effectiveness on anger management.

## What is CBT?

According to reliable sources, cognitive-behavioral therapy came to light in the 1960s. CBT came into existence with the help of a psychoanalyst of the University of Pennsylvania Medical School, namely Aaron Beck. He tried to look for an experimental or observational basis for those psychoanalysis treatments which were utilized for depression. During his attempt, he was unable to find any such basis, but one thing that came to light was that cognition played an important part in depression. Thus, Beck founded or was the first person to conceptualize cognitive-behavioral therapy. It has proved its efficiency as a useful treatment choice for a wide range of psychological issues such as anxiety disorders, depression, uncontrolled anger, acute mental illness, eating and sleeping disorders, drug and alcohol use problems, schizophrenia, etc.

Innumerable research studies state that CBT or cognitive-behavioral therapy directs to great improvement in both the quality and functioning of life. This time-sensitive talk therapy is helpful in identifying and coping with particular challenges rapidly. CBT requires fewer sessions than any other form of therapy as well as it is performed in a well-planned way. This therapy leads to solving the present problems as well as teaches skills to the clients for modifying dysfunctional behavior and thinking. CBT is performed on the basis of the concept that an individual's feelings, thoughts, physical actions, and sensations are all connected to each other, and negative feelings and thoughts can trap him/her in a ferocious cycle.

The aim of CBT is to assist you in dealing with problems related to uncontrolled anger in a positive manner. It is done by breaking down the problems into smaller fragments. Unlike various other talk therapies, cognitive-behavioral therapy focuses on a person's current problems. It does not deal with past issues. It utilizes a variety of practical ways to improve the mental state or condition on a regular basis. CBT teaches you to use the anger management skills that you came across while pursuing the therapy in your regular life.

During the CBT session, a proficient therapist encourages the person who has come up for anger management to speak up about his or her feelings and thoughts as well as the things that are giving trouble to him/her. A lot of people do exist who find it difficult to reveal their feelings openly in front of their therapist. But, there is nothing to worry about at all as your therapist will surely assist you in gaining comfort and more confidence.

The sessions are done either on one is to one basis or along with the affected person's family members. Your therapist might require a certain number of sessions for understanding your present concerns and the situation entirely. One of the basic facts that a therapist of cognitive-behavioral therapy needs to analyze is the causes of why his or her client is unable to control anger. Knowing the specific reasons or situations behind such outbursts of emotion is highly necessary for proceeding with the treatment.

Cognitive-behavioral therapy possesses a firm goal. Its goal is to make people understand and teach them that no matter how hard they try, they won't ever be able to control every single aspect of this world. But, that does not mean you have to get angry whenever you find anything not happening in the way you wanted it to be. CBT will help you to manage your anger, no matter how messy the situation is. This anger management therapy will teach you various ways of interpreting and dealing with the different types of things in their environment.

You might find it difficult in the beginning, but gradually you will get hold of your anger by pursuing this therapy. Thus, you may say that CBT is very much helpful in managing anger. It even assists those people who suffer from specific kinds of emotional hardships that do not need psychotropic medication. You will definitely be very glad to know that the affordability of CBT is more than various other kinds of talk therapy. Another benefit of CBT is helping clients to develop the skills of coping up with anger. Such skills prove to be helpful both at present as well as in the future days.

## Types of CBT

Cognitive-behavioral therapy includes a vast range of approaches and methods that address emotions, behaviors, as well as thoughts. The techniques may range from materials of self-help to structured psychotherapists. Various forms of therapeutic approaches are there that are associated with CBT.

- DBT or dialectical behavior therapy – This particular therapy addresses behaviors and thoughts while combining strategies like mindfulness and emotional regulation.

- Cognitive therapy – The main aim of cognitive therapy is to identify as well as alter distorted or inaccurate thinking patterns, behaviors, emotional responses, and a lot more. Analyzing a person's sudden and awkward behavior after he or she gets angry is an essential part of this therapy.

- REBT or rational emotive behavior therapy – This form of cognitive-behavioral therapy involves the identification of irrational or, you may say, absurd beliefs. After identifying them properly, the next or final step is to learn recognizing as well as changing such thought patterns.

- Multimodal therapy – Now, this therapy states that any type of psychological problems, be it anger or depression, must be handled by giving effort to seven different yet interconnected procedures. Some of the modalities include sensation, behavior, imagery, affect interpersonal factors, cognition, biological, or drug considerations.

Every single form of CBT or cognitive-behavioral therapy proceeds with a distinct approach. Even if the approaches are different, yet all of them are meant for dealing with the hidden thought patterns due to which psychological sufferings are caused.

Certain core principles do exist on the basis of which cognitive-behavioral therapy is carried out successfully. Some of the principles include:

- Psychological issues are based partly on unhelpful or faulty thinking processes.

- Psychological issues are also based partly on learned arrangements of non-cooperating or unhelpful behavior.

- Individuals who suffer from various psychological problems have the capability of learning improved or developed means of coping with them. They even become more practical and efficient in their own lives slowly. Besides this, they also attain the ability to control weird or aggressive behaviors caused due to anger.

Treatment for managing anger with the assistance of CBT involves various efforts for changing a person's thinking patterns. Such strategies may include:

- Utilizing skills for solving problems so that difficult situations can be handled effectively

- Achieving a better way of understanding the reason behind the opposite person's behavior and also realizing the motivation of other people

- Learn developing an excellent sense of being confident in almost all situations

The treatment procedure of CBT also involves certain efforts for changing a person's behavioral patterns. Now, these strategies or efforts may include:

- Facing the things that an individual is afraid of and stop avoiding them

- Learning effective skills of relaxing one's body as well as calming the mind even in tough situations

- Utilizing role play for the preparation of problematic interaction with other people

It is not necessary that all the different types of cognitive-behavioral therapy will make use of all the above-mentioned strategies. Rather, both the client and the therapist work in a co-operative fashion. They work together to develop a better understanding of all the problems as well as for developing the best strategy of treatment. This therapy assists individuals in learning ways so that they can become their very own therapists.

## Length of the Therapy

Usually, CBT is considered to be a therapy that requires a short term. The term ranges from about 5-20 sessions. Each session lasts for approximately thirty minutes to one hour. Your therapist will discuss with you the number of sessions required by you. Some of the factors that need to be considered include:

- The severity of the symptoms

- Type of situation or disorder

- The time that an individual is requiring for making progress

- The amount of stress that the person is experiencing

- The amount of support received from the family members as well as other close ones

## Things That Happen During the Sessions of CBT

First of all, when the sessions are going on, you will be expected to work together with your experienced therapist for breaking down all the problems that you face into separate parts, like your physical actions, feelings, and thoughts. Both the client and the therapist try analyzing these specific areas in order to understand whether they are unhelpful or unrealistic. It even helps in determining the effects that those areas have on you.

It is then that your therapist will get an opportunity of helping you to work out the ways of changing such behaviors and thoughts that are unhelpful by nature. After giving efforts on the things that you can alter, you will be instructed by your therapist to practice the required changes in real life. In your next session, you will be asked by your therapist to discuss or narrate the experience that you acquired while practicing the changes.

The clients are given to practice various positive exercises in between the sessions. They are also provided with certain homework exercises that they are expected to perform in between the sessions. Homework activities may include the regular reading of novels or other storybooks. Your therapist may also ask you to maintain a journal of your regular activities. In some cases, you may also be instructed to do certain activities that are outside or different from your basic therapy sessions. By doing so, clients learn to develop various coping skills. Such skills help them in changing their way of thinking, problematic emotions, as well as undesired and, at the same time, odd behaviors.

CBT aims to teach you ways of applying those skills that you got to learn while pursuing the treatment in your regular life. This will surely assist you in managing the problems that you face because of uncontrolled anger as well as prevent them from having a negative effect on your personal and professional life also after the course of your treatment finishes.

If you are willing to get the best results of cognitive-behavioral therapy for managing your anger, then it is your duty to be honest and open during the sessions of your treatment. This therapy becomes more effective when you participate actively and share all the problems that you face openly with your therapist. The success rate depends on the client's willingness to share his/her thoughts, experiences, and feelings. Many people lack motivation or feel down during the sessions of cognitive-behavioral therapy. You must be prepared as it may happen to you too. Many-a-times, you may also feel like skipping the upcoming therapy sessions. But, you need to control this particular temptation of yours. The reason behind this is that if by chance you skip any of the sessions of the therapy, then your progress may get disrupted. Thus, you need to make up your mind that no matter what happens and how much negative or restless feeling you get from within, you won't give up in between the proceedings of the treatment. Talk to your therapist if you get any such feeling as he/she will motivate you to stick firmly to the treatment plan.

A lot of people do exist who hold a belief that they will get to see positive and instant results just after going through one or two sessions. But, to be very honest, this belief is not at all true. You need to understand the fact that working on issues that have an emotional background can prove to be painful, as well as requires a huge amount of hard work. It is quite common to get a worse feeling in the initial stages of the therapy because you have to confront your current problems. Thus, you need to make up your mind that several sessions may be required, and only after that will you get to notice improvements.

Now, if you want to experience the benefit of this particular therapy, then you need to consult with or seek assistance from a proficient physician or behavioral therapist. He/she is the best person who will be able to guide you in the best possible way of managing or controlling anger.

# 7.
# Cognitive Distortions That Fuel Anger and How to Deal With Them?

Outbursts of anger are not fate's decree. Not only can anger outbursts be managed, but they can also be drastically minimized and can be controlled. Anger, which is self-directed, is generally thought to be problematic and can cause bitterness, which can result in feelings of sadness and guilt. On the other hand, anger that is directed towards other people is considered to be healthier since the individual gains their relief by unloading their anger, which refreshes and vents their feelings. In reality, however, the relief that comes after one's anger release doesn't last for a long time.

A majority of people truly believe that their anger roots in the actions of other people. Anger is, in fact, built in our minds, and it develops because of how they interpret other people's actions. It is wrong to think that people around you have the power to make us angry. Your emotions are not a result of a particular event, but rather they are the result of the meaning that you give to that event.

One of the major reasons for anger is cognitive distortions. Cognitive distortions can be described as habitual errors in thinking. Such patterns of thoughts cause people to see reality in a distorted and negative way. People tend to experience cognitive distortions quite often. However, if they occur too often, they could also cause relationship problems, deepen depression, increase anxiety, as well as result in several other complications. Studies have shown that people tend to develop cognitive disorders as a coping mechanism to deal with adverse life events. Life adversity can result in behavioral and emotional problems, among other things. If those adverse events get more severe and prolonged, it's more likely that the individual can develop one or more cognitive distortions. One study also suggested that people have developed cognitive distortions as an evolutionary method of survival. This means that stress could have made individuals change their methods of thinking so that it becomes useful to them for their survival at the moment. However, these kinds of thoughts are irrational and unhealthy in the long term.

## Types of Cognitive Distortions

In 1979, Emery, Shaw, Rush, and Beck conducted a study on cognitive distortions and revealed that there are at least ten different kinds of distorted thinking patterns. Dr. David Burns, a pioneer on cognitive behavior therapy, mentioned these in his 1999 bestseller 'The Feeling Good Handbook.' Cognitive behavior therapy (CBT) is a method by which cognitive distortions can be identified and used to treat several issues, including eating disorders, anxiety, addiction, as well as depression.

Here are some kinds of cognitive distortions that can fuel anger:

### All or Nothing Thinking

All or nothing thinking is a kind of cognitive distortive thinking pattern that is very common in people suffering from anxiety-related issues like depression, panic disorder, etc. People tend to divide their views into two extremes when they are thinking in terms of all or nothing. Everything – from their life experiences to their views about themselves – is split into just black and white. This leaves little or no space for areas that fall in between the two. This kind of thinking involves the use of absolute terms like 'ever' or 'never' as well as an inability to see the solutions to any problem or the alternatives in any situation. In the case of people suffering from depression and anxiety, they, therefore, see only the downside of any situation. Individuals who fall victim to this kind of cognitive distortion start believing that they are either successful in life or an absolute failure. Individuals who have frequent panic attacks are also susceptible to this kind of distortion.

They view themselves as inadequate or unworthy and might also ignore how valuable they are in other roles, like that of a parent, employee, or friend.

Rather than trying to find a middle ground, people with all or nothing pattern of thinking think in extremes. This can also lead to relapses. For instance, let's consider David, who feels like a failure because he can't get sober despite his efforts. Every time she messes up, he drinks to intoxication, thinking that she has already failed anyway instead of acknowledging that he made an error in judgment and trying to move on from it.

## Overgeneralization

Individuals suffering from anxiety or depression are frequently affected by overgeneralization. This cognitive distortion can worsen their fear, depression, and anxiety. They tend to apply a single experience to all their experiences, including those that are going to happen in the future. For instance, when you have a bad experience in one relationship and start thinking that you are simply bad at relationships. Or, you score low in a particular math test and develop a belief that you are simply hopeless at the subject in general.

Using words like 'everyone,' 'nobody,' 'always,' and 'never' can make any problem look larger than they actually are. Overgeneralization also makes an occasional experience feel like an insufferable and ongoing event. Exaggeration is not always the entire truth. One of the best ways to overcome overgeneralization is by making a true effort to search for exceptions. When you start understanding that different people behave in different ways, it can make their actions a little less upsetting. It is ideal to clearly describe specific situations and avoid using generalized terms as much as you can. You will start to overgeneralize if you think in terms of only black and white. This dichotomous method of thinking tends to result in anger when others behave in a way that seems less than perfect to you. One method of dealing with this is by practicing searching for the grey. Try using qualifying adverbs and adjectives like 'somewhat,' 'a lot,' 'a little,' etc.

You can also try to see other people as contradictory, confusing, and complex beings. If you take a closer look at the person you are angry at, you might be surprised to see that you also like some of their personality traits.

## Labeling

Labeling is a type of cognitive distortion that involves making sweeping judgments that are negative and often inflammatory. People tend to generalize other people or themselves by taking a single characteristic and applying it to the entire person. For example, if someone talked to you in a rude way, you label him as a jerk; you label someone as irresponsible because she is frequently late to work, or you might label yourself as a failure because you failed a single test.

When people engage in labeling, they tend to describe the whole person instead of thinking more objective about their behavior. Because of this, they filter out all the other information that doesn't fall under the label that they have assigned to the person and see the whole person through that label. They start believing it more as the label starts to feel like a more proper description of the person.

As a cognitive disorder, labeling can fuel and maintain painful emotions in addition to causing inaccurate thinking. It could fuel your anger by turning the other person's behavior into a worthless object. For example, someone who spoke to you rudely might not be a bad person or a jerk. He could just be in a rush at that moment. It could also be that the person just speaks directly and is a very kind and generous person in reality. It's almost always inaccurate to make a single broad assumption on the basis of one or a few isolated data points. That's why labeling is wrong. Inaccurate thinking can also trigger feelings of hopelessness, despair, sadness, etc. If you label yourself as a failure after merely failing a test, you won't be able to solve the problem.

Being specific is one of the best ways to combat labeling. Concentrate on the behavior you find annoying and define it as accurately as you can. How did the other person's behavior affect you? What happened? How often does it happen? When did it happen? These kinds of questions don't involve making derogatory comments regarding the other person or making judgments about the person.

## Personalization and Blame

This is one of the most damaging and self-destructive forms of cognitive distortion that fuels anger. People having this kind of cognitive distortion tend to put the entire blame for an event on yourself or someone else. People start believing that other people are purposefully doing bad things to them and that they won't let them get away with it.

Often without having any evidence, you start believing that the other person's actions and statements are directed towards you, and you start feeling personally attacked. You overlook your own role in a situation and redefine the problem so as to put the blame on the other person. Even though blaming other people might make you feel good at times, it also tends to leave you feeling helpless. You lose your power and ability to change the situation; that's the source of your pain if you start blaming other people.

If you try to remember that the people around you are also trying to do their best, it can help you deal with your anger. Remember that everyone generally behaves in a manner that suits their personal requirements. Similarly, the person you are blaming might also be doing whatever they think will help them take care of themselves.

## Mental Filter

Mental filtering is another common cognitive distortion that a majority of people do from time to time. It is the opposite of overgeneralization, but it also has the same negative outcome. It involves filtering out the positives regarding a particular person or event and focusing only on the negatives. Therefore, similar to a drop of ink that has the ability to discolor a glass of water, your perception of the other person also darkens. You ignore all the positive things that the other person has done and their good intentions and concentrate only on what he or she has done to upset you.

Mental filtering is often accompanied by extremely high expectations, which involve always doing something in a perfect way. All efforts are judged against the standard of perfection. If you fulfill those standards, it will seem like you are simply doing what's expected. However, it will get very easy to ignore all of your successes if you fall short even occasionally, and then you will start to concentrate only on the few occasions where you were unsuccessful.

Focusing only on the negatives can result in unhealthy pessimism, poor self-esteem, and depressed mood. One of the key things that you can do when you think you are participating in this kind of cognitive distortion is to review the actual evidence present in front of you.

## Catastrophizing

This kind of cognitive distortion involves more than simply making things worse than they are or making a mountain out of a molehill. It involves the tendency to imagine the worst possible scenario for just a bad situation, to take a bad thing, and run with it. You set yourself up to reply in a hostile or angry way when you magnify things and start viewing them as horrendous, terrible, or awful. You might start acting as if your exaggerated or distorted view of the occasion was the true fact. For example, suppose an expected paycheck hasn't arrived in the mail. An individual who catastrophizes will start to think that the paycheck will never reach him, as a result of which he won't be able to pay his rent and will get evicted.

Even though it's easy to view this thinking distortion as a hilarious over-reaction, individuals might have developed it as a result of repeated adverse events (such as childhood traumas or chronic pain) so often that they start thinking the worst in every situation. Luckily there are also methods by which they can control this distortion. Firstly, they need to create a realistic assessment and be honest in their answers. Secondly, describe their situation in a very precise language, and lastly, they need to look at the entire picture and not just the moment that annoyed them. There are positives and negatives in every relationship and every situation. You can neutralize your anger by focusing on the positives.

## Tips For Dealing With Cognitive Distortions

- **Thinking in the shades of grey** – Try to see the gray area or the middle ground instead of letting yourself think in extremes. You could rate how you are feeling on a scale of one to hundred, with a hundred being the best and one being the worst. Soon you will begin to see that only some events are a hundred or a one. Thus, most of the events are not as extreme as you might think they are.

- **Analyzing the cost and benefit** – The practice of analyzing the cost and benefit seeks the answer to one key question: are your cognitive distortions hurting or helping you? By examining the benefits and drawbacks of your distortive thinking patterns, you can easily understand that your cognitive distortions are a limited framework with which you can examine any situation. After that, you might become more disposed to re-evaluate and overcome them. Therefore, create a list of pros and cons and then challenge and reevaluate them.

- **Mindfulness** – The practice of mindfulness is quite simple. It is the practice of being aware of the present moment. It can help decrease obsessive thinking or rumination and also help calm the mind. Through intentional breathing, body scanning, and focused awareness, mindfulness can help bring your mind back to reality when distortive thoughts blow things out of proportion in your mind.

- **Survey method** – You can try finding some perspective by surveying or consulting your loved ones or your trusted friends. At times you will be able to understand your cognitive distortions in a better way if you discuss how you are feeling with the people you love and trust. You can also have the ones you trust to tell you the truth.

- **Journaling** – Writing down your feelings in a journal is a cathartic and powerful method of expressing the emotions you are feeling at the moment. In addition to that, it is also a great way of distinguishing the kind of cognitive distortive pattern you are engaging in so that you can figure out your next step in a logical manner. You will also have a complete repository of thoughts with you once you have been journaling for long enough. Thus, you can check your progress over time, which could help you identify and replace any negative thought patterns that might be stopping you from reaching your full potential.

- **Opinion or fact challenge** – Jot down what you are feeling at the current moment on a sheet of paper. Then, go one by one and examine whether your beliefs is either an opinion or a fact. Try to be candid and honest with yourself. Always remember that opinions are deeply-rooted in personal beliefs, while facts are objectively true. Thus, opinions might or might not be applicable to other people.

# 8.
# How to Communicate When You Are Angry?

You must have heard this many times in various different situations, but it is true that communication is indeed the key to a lot of problems. You will be surprised to know how much help honest communication can bring. Be it verbal or written, communicating with someone can bring out our honest thoughts, which, if not expressed properly, can cause serious damage. For people who have anger management issues, it is highly recommended to communicate in whichever way they seem fit so that they might receive help soon, and the underlying problem might not escalate and that the process of healing might become easier.

## Try Not Venting Out Your Anger

Venting out your cooped-up anger might seem like a great idea. It might feel like a very necessary relief when the anger inside you is taking a toll on your behavior otherwise. But research has shown that venting out might not be a good idea after all. It doesn't have the desired effect. On the other hand, it escalates the problem. It reinforces all the negative emotions that had caused the anger, thereby instigating further negativity in you.

The next thing to be kept in mind is the person you are venting out to. A person might choose a friend or a colleague, or a very trusted family member for this purpose. He, in his angry and flustered state, will go and tell his story that his making him lose his temper. The most basic response to this will be them telling a similar story in order to pacify him by giving in to his thoughts at that moment. Now, what does that tell about the position of these people in his life? What is the result of such an exchange? For that moment, it might seem the right thing to do, and hence we might choose to do that often. But this makes the other person hugely uncomfortable as they might not know what the correct thing to do is, and at the same time, it does nothing to solve the problem or give any constructive measures to keep that anger in check. What it does is to only pacify the situation for the time being.

It is very understandable that, as humans, we need to talk to someone about how and what we feel. Thus, a good and honest conversation is always encouraged. But the basic difference between having a conversation and venting out is that the former is a two-sided encounter while the latter is predominantly a one-sided angry exchange. But just because we can vent out doesn't mean we should. Neither will it stop the same situation from happening again in the future, nor is it good for our health.

## Try Not to Communicate Aggressively But Assertively

One of the most important things is to take a pause and look back on one's own behavior and to not repeat the mistake if found any. The difference between aggression and assertion will become a bit clearer. Anger, when asserted in the correct direction, can be constructive, as opposed to aggression. There are few very basic questions that a person can ask oneself in such a situation that might be of help.

- *Firstly*, ask yourself what it is that you wish to achieve in that angry state of mind. If it is the solution to the situation that you want, then talking it out calmly is the best option. But if you don't care about any of that because your anger is not letting you think straight, then that is a problem.

- *Secondly*, the key to communicating in an assertive manner is to let the other person know clearly what, according to you, went wrong and what is it exactly that you would like to change in the future. That will take the misunderstandings out of the way, making way for a transparent exchange. Not beating around the bush will make the other person understand your viewpoint better.

- *Thirdly*, ask yourself what you wish to achieve after you have that conversation. Do you really want to have a solution to that problem, or was that conversation just a means to have a one-to-one with that other person? You need to think twice if it is the latter.

- *Fourthly,* ask yourself how you want to feel inside once you have had a conversation with the person. You might feel that you now have a better understanding of the situation and of the other person once you have talked it out, or you might also feel that by talking, you gave in to your vulnerabilities, and that might be embarrassing for you. One needs to clear out these doubts in order to take the next step forward.

- *Fifthly,* the key to having an assertive conversation and to not let it turn into an aggressive one is to keep in mind to let one's focus be on the problem at hand that has caused the anger, rather than focusing on the other person with whom the misunderstanding has started. You need to realize that it is not the problem against whom you have a personal vendetta. Finding a solution to that problem is the key and not bringing harm to the other person.

- *Lastly,* the thing that needs to be kept in mind as you are having the conversation is that no matter what the problem is, you need to keep a civil tone and a respectful attitude throughout. Shouting will only intensify the tension unnecessarily, making the conversation lose its desired purpose. The message will get lost among all the hullabaloo, and let's be honest – nobody likes being shouted at. You wouldn't want the same thing happening to you, so don't do it to someone else.

## Practice Writing About Your Feelings Instead of Speaking

This can be a really beneficial alternative to communicate when you are angry if you find speaking to be a problem. Writing out your honest feelings can have many benefits. As you start writing, your thoughts tend to become clearer. So, you can analyze properly within yourself as to exactly where does the problem lies. This gives you much-needed clarity, which will help you to communicate better. Writing helps you build a structure upon which you can build your thoughts.

As you start emptying your mind on the paper, you basically empty your stress. As you start seeing the entire issue with a much more practical mindset, you learn to rationalize your feelings and actions. Writing about your honest feelings also makes you learn a lot about yourself, which will help you take responsible actions in the future. Gaining an awareness of your reality helps you revitalize psychologically.

As you let your negativities go, you tend to become a much happier person, who will be more focused on finding the solution for the problem rather than getting revenge. Many times, speaking in a fit of anger might not be able to convey what you actually want to put out there. You might also say things you don't mean to and regret it later. Writing reduces such possibilities.

## Improve Your Vocabulary to Express Your Feelings Better

The majority of the time, a conversation doesn't take the desired turn because one or both the concerned parties are not able to communicate properly. The situation worsens if, during an angry fit, people fail to express themselves properly, more so because, at times, people might not have the proper vocabulary. As a result, they settle for generalized statements which in no way convey the actual sentiments. Misunderstandings can further increase due to this. A person might also be of the habit of going out of the line while talking; as a result, both the parties might completely forget what the actual issue was. Hence it is extremely important to know what are the keys to an effective conversation while you are angry to have the desired effect and impact. There are few ways in which this can be done –

- *Try staying focused on what you want to say* – It is very much possible that your anger makes you forget what you actually wanted to say. Many factors could be responsible for this. You might not like the other person at all, and hence having a conversation with him might be unpleasant. Your emotions can get the better of you, and hence you might not be able to form coherent thoughts. Your anger might make you become violent in some extreme cases. In such cases, knowing what to say becomes really beneficial. Your vocabulary will do the work that your actions can't. Using the correct words have the greatest impact during times when other methods are not in use. Suitable vocabulary will save you from being misguided by blind rage.

- *Try not to stretch the issue unnecessarily* – During the initial days of learning to manage your anger, one of the most challenging things that one might face is to express what one is feeling in a constructive way. The trick basically is to keep your vocation to the point and not rant about it to others all the time. The other person is likely to get irritated if the same thing is repeated again and again. After the brain reaches that saturation point, it simply stops registering more information. So, if a person keeps reiterating the same point, again and again, the chances are that the other person will simply stop paying any heed to it and will start ignoring that person.

Keeping this in mind is extremely important that you should take deep breaths and proper pauses while having a conversation because when you are angry, this practice will especially help you keep your calm, remember what you intend to say in the correct way, and will also make the other person realize that you actually mean what you say.

## Understand That it is More Important How You Are Saying Something Rather Than What You Are Saying

Try and understand that if you have a heated argument with somebody who has gone up to the point where you alone or you both are shouting at each other, in all probability, none of you are actually listening to what the other person is saying. All the main concerns of the discussion are actually not making any sense, and the entire effort in basically going in vain. So, it is extremely important to put forth your views in a sophisticated way that will actually reach the other person without heightening the tension. Hence how you are saying becomes more important than what you are saying. Now there are certain ways, which, if kept in mind, will make having meaningful communication easier.

- *The pace of talking-* You will notice that the speed of your speech tends to invariably increase when you are angry and trying to have a conversation because, quite naturally, you are trying to say many things at once. At times you might also feel that you are not speaking as fast as you want to. Try not to do this. Remember that whatever you have to say will only have its desired impact if the other actually understands it. You running with your speech will only have the opposite effect. So, try giving appropriate pauses between your words to make it more comprehensible.

- *The volume of your speech-* Remember that the volume you use during a conversation is very important to convey the mood of the conversation. While on one side, a very soft voice with your meek and mild disposition might make the other person not take you seriously, on the other hand, an extremely loud voice with you shouting violently will make the other person cower away from you without actually listening. The key, therefore, is to take up an attitude that falls in between these two. Your voice should be loud without being screaming. Your speech should be clear and not incomprehensible so that it might sound responsible. Your words should be respectful, and your attitude should be sophisticated.

## Take Professional Help to Manage Anger

The inability to manage your anger can really become a serious problem if not given its due importance, as a prolonged habit of keeping this suppressed might lead to various psychological and health problems. Taking constructive steps towards anger management is, of course, advisable. But if it goes out of hand, then seeking professional help is advisable. That will give you a positive push towards managing your emotions and thereby communicate better and help you lead a better and independent life. Talking to a therapist might help you see things objectively and help change your thoughts and behavior for the better. You will learn how to react to situations better.

CBT, also known as Cognitive Behavioural Therapy, can help you form a healthy relationship with your own self by managing your stress and locating your source of anger. It will help to locate your trigger points and teach you to deal with them. It will also help you to understand the other person's perspective, helping to clear away the misunderstandings. You will learn to take charge of your situation and will also learn about the best ways to communicate with others during that time.

## Take a Deep Breath

This is probably the easiest thing to do, which takes the most effort. Every time you are angry, and you feel that you might actually lose control if you try and communicate with someone at that point, take a pause, and then take a deep breath. Ask yourself how prepared are you to conduct a conversation. If your brain is giving you any red signals, then it is best to calm down first and talk about it sometime later. After all, not getting worked up is the intention. You might start facing health issues otherwise from too much stress. On the other hand, if you feel that you are in control of the situation, then definitely go ahead with the conversation.

In conclusion, always remember that you are not a rouge. Getting angry is a very natural thing, and it happens to everyone. Wanting a conversation to find a solution for it is the correct thing to do. So, you are not doing anything wrong by conducting such an interaction. The only thing that needs to be kept in mind is that as human beings, we are prone to make mistakes of which we are not proud of. So, it is best to take precautionary measures when we have the time to do it. If we keep in mind the basic few steps that are mentioned above, then communicating with others, even when you are angry, shouldn't be any trouble. On the contrary, you will be able to effectively conduct your energy towards something constructive. That being said, also remember that anger management is easier said than done. So don't beat yourself up for it, and please give yourself some time.

# 9.
# Tips For Managing Conflicts For People With Anger Issues

Anger issues are a serious problem that needs to be dealt with in a proper way to avoid worse situations. Let us discuss more on this.

## Why Do Conflicts Happen?

Human beings are complicated, and so are their reasons for conflict. The reasons vary from person to person. Conflicts between two people arise only when there is a pre-existing relationship between them. Conflicts may also arise between strangers, and these conflicts are mainly circumstantial, and nobody is emotionally invested in these. When we engage in some sort of conflict with a stranger, we may feel angry and frustrated, but it doesn't affect us emotionally. The conflicts that truly affect us are the ones which we have with those who matter to us, i.e., our family members, friends, loved ones, etc. If we have a conflict with a close person and keep the conflict unresolved, it will affect us tremendously in the long run.

Every kind of relationship faces conflict at some time or the other. It doesn't necessarily mean that things won't work out, or the relationship is not worth it. Conflicts are normal, and they need to be resolved in order to maintain a healthy relationship with people. It is very important to know about the causes that are mainly responsible for causing conflicts. Although they vary to a large degree from people to people, let us discuss some of the common causes that are known to cause conflicts between people.

- *Different desires, goals, or agendas* – This is a very common reason for conflict. The difference in desires and goals may be as simple as choosing where to eat and as complicated as to where to live. Opinions, agendas, priorities vary from person to person, and when a person tries to impose theirs on others, that is when the conflict arises. In these kinds of conflicts, one of the parties gives in and tries to resolve the situation, but you need to understand that it is not resolving anything. Giving in or compromising every time doesn't end the conflicts; it just increases the chances of future conflicts.

- *Having something that someone else needs* – Suppose you need something that your friend has. You go and ask for that thing from him, and he refuses. Even after repetitive requests, he turns you down. You are most likely to feel agitated. This is not just annoying for you but for your friend too. You are thinking, why is he not being generous and thoughtful, whereas he is thinking, why are you not going and buying the thing you need instead of continuously bothering him. In situations like this, none of the parties are necessarily right or wrong. They just have different opinions and views, which the other one finds hard to accept. Conflicts are likely to arise in situations like these.

- *Personalities* – The conflicts arising from varied personalities are a little sensitive. All individuals have their own unique personalities, and that is what distinguishes them from each other. Sometimes this personality is the main factor that contributes to creating tension between two people. Suppose you have a friend who likes to be in the center of attention always. You find him cracking jokes on you often to make people laugh and attract the eyes. You may find it embarrassing and awkward to listen to jokes made about you and your personal life. You may feel agitated and tell him not to do that. He, on the other hand, can't even understand why you are being so paranoid about it and just blows you off and continue making jokes about you. This is something that can give rise to conflicts. These kinds of conflicts don't arise between strangers. They only arise between people who know each other for a long time.

- *A significant change* – When a significant change brings significant changes in your lifestyle, conflicts are likely to arise. Suppose your partner got a promotion. You are happy for his success, but your happiness may be short-lived. You will start to feel weird when you see certain changes occurring because of that. Your partner has started spending more hours at the office and comes home late. You'll see that he always stays stressed and rarely takes part in family activities. You may adjust at the beginning, but slowly you are likely to lose patience and burst out. You may feel that it is unfair on your part, and you are deprived somehow, whereas your partner will feel agitated at you for not appreciating his or her hard work. He or she will be clueless as to why you are so upset and making a big deal out of it. In this situation, none of you are right or wrong. It is just that when we see a slight change in things that we are used to doing or getting, we tend to lose our minds because of it. This is the reason why conflicts occur when there is a significant change. Some examples of the causes of these kinds of conflicts are – extramarital affair, child's new college, a new girlfriend or a boyfriend, engagement, weight gain or loss, illness, career success, losing a job, etc.

- *Betrayal* – This is one thing that is bound to cause conflicts. If you get betrayed by someone, you will lash out at that person no matter what. Suppose you share a secret with your friend asking her not to tell that to anybody. The next day if you hear that thing from someone else's mouth, you are more likely to doubt your friend first. It may or may not be true that your friend is guilty of disclosing the matter. But it is surely a matter of conflict. Being dishonest, playing mind games, cheating, stealing, and not being honest about something are some of the common causes for the conflict of betrayal.

- *Irresponsible behavior* – If you see that you are the only one who takes care of all the responsibilities, then one day, it is likely to make you lash out. Responsibilities should always be shared. It is nobody's sole duty to be responsible and take care of everything. Irresponsible behavior from your spouse, friends, or family is what makes you on edge. You tend to feel angry and frustrated as to why you are the only one responsible for doing all the work. When you try to communicate this with your partner, he or she might not be able to understand your side because they never actually felt it. So, this may lead to a huge conflict. Some common causes for these kinds of conflicts are – canceling plans, passing weird comments about other people's looks and appearances, never returning a borrowed item, repeatedly forgetting anniversaries and birthdays, etc.

## What is Conflict Resolution?

Conflict resolution is the method of solving problems and resolving them for finding a peaceful solution.

## Reduce Stress

You must have supportive relationships in your life for maintaining both physical and mental health. The best way to deal with a conflict is to eliminate that person forever from your life. In case the person is someone important, and you are unable to do that, there are some other techniques too.

- Try to have neutral conversations. Make sure to avoid discussing things that cause tension like politics, religion, etc. If you notice that the person you are talking to is repeatedly trying to pull you into a conversation, which you know can have adverse effects. If you don't feel like conversing with anybody, then just carry on with yourselves.

- Try to accept their real selves. When you are dealing with people who are difficult to handle, don't even try to change them. If you do, you are more likely to invite criticism, cause defensiveness, or can even get you into a power struggle. When you do this, you become a more difficult person to deal with.

- You should never let your partner say or do bad things to you, even if you get hurt from that. Stop compromising and adjusting to everything that is happening around you. You need to know about the things you can take control over and the things you have a say in. So, once you start taking your own stand, conflicts are less likely to happen.

- Conflicts don't usually occur because one person is bad. It generally occurs because of the unhealthy patterns of interaction between two people. If you work on changing your response and start responding in a healthier way, it will reduce the conflicts too.

- Try to focus on the positive side of the person you are

interacting with. Every person has a good and a bad side. If you continuously keep noticing the bad side of a person, you are going to have conflicts with that person forever. To avoid this, try to focus on that person's good side. If you do this, that person will feel adored and appreciated, and your conflict will be resolved automatically.

- Make sure to always remember the person you are dealing with. Focusing on a person's good side doesn't mean completely disregarding their bad side. Focus on their good side but also keep their traits and characteristics in your mind. Don't expect love and affection from a person incapable of giving it, or rely on a person who isn't trustworthy, or share your secrets with a person who likes to gossip. Accept them for who they are and then behave accordingly.

- Always make sure to get support. Meet your needs from others who are capable of doing that. For example – share your secrets with a friend who is trustworthy, or start writing to express your thoughts, opinions, and desires. You can even seek professional help and consult a psychiatrist. This will ensure to remove the existing weight off of your relationship, and now it is all gone. This will make sure that you and the other person to remove a source of conflict.

- It is very important to know when to leave. It is okay to put efforts to try and mend things, but there is a threshold to everything. Know when it is time to leave. If the other person remains consistently abusive and inconsiderate towards you, it is wiser of you to just cut all the ties with that person and move on.

## Control Your Emotions

When you are in the middle of a tensed conversation, you are most likely to get emotionally worked up as well. Conflicts may often seem like threats because you feel like your actions or viewpoints are in question, and your body gets worked up and ready to fight. This triggers your sympathetic nervous system. This will stop you from thinking rationally, and you will do irrational things because of that.

There are some ways in which you can control your emotions.

- Breathe frequently. In tensed situations, simple mindfulness techniques are the biggest saviors. When you feel that the situation is getting tensed and out of hands, try to divert your focus to your breathing. Notice the feeling of air passing through your nose and passing out. This will help you to divert your attention and will make sure that you stay centered. You can even try counting your breaths, as suggested by some experts.

- Make sure to focus on your own body. While having a difficult conversation, if you sit still, you will just be stacking the disappointments within yourself. Some experts say that walking around and standing up helps in activating the part of your brain responsible for rational thinking. When you are in a sitting arrangement with that person, you may feel a little awkward to suddenly get up and walk, but you can at least make use of these mindfulness exercises to stay away from conflicts as much as possible.

- Start acknowledging and labeling your feelings. When you give too much attention to your feelings and thoughts, your brain gets pre-occupied and takes away your sense of rationality. Labeling will help you to see what your feelings and thoughts actually are.

- Try taking a break sometimes. If you give yourself time to analyze a particular situation, then you are likely to stay away from tense situations. This is because your mind got a lot of time to analyze all the things to be able to make rational decisions again.

- Always remember that you are not the only one who is supposed to be in trouble. Your counterpart may also be facing some troubles and tragedies. Sometimes you should take a step back and let the other person vent out their anger and frustration. So, if you continue to have a conversation in this state, then it will do you no good. Sometimes, it is important to take a step back and wait for things to fall into place again.

## Work on Your Nonverbal Communication Skills

When you are in the middle of a conflict, your non-verbal behavior (certain body movements) says a lot about how you feel and what you mean to the other person. Certain non-verbal behaviors are good in grim situations, but some of them are definitely not. For example, if someone says that they agree with you while rolling their eyes, will you be convinced that they agree with you? Obviously not! Although he said they agree, still his non-verbal behavior clearly portrayed that he was saying those in a mocking way and not in a literal way. Studies have shown that the majority of people believe what they understand from the other person's non-verbal behavior than what they say from their mouths. Studies have shown that when a person is involved in a conflict situation, he or she becomes more attentive towards the other person's body language. This makes it more important to check your non-verbal communication when you are involved in a conflict. Try to pay attention to your body language as well as the other person's body language. When the other person says something, try to maintain a facial expression expressing genuine interest. Also, try to maintain a calm voice. These will help you to take control of the situation before it worsens.

## Make Careful Use of Humor

Humor helps you to interrupt the power struggle. It instantly eases the tension between you two and helps you to reconnect with that person. It makes you spontaneous. Laughter can change your ways of behaving and thinking. You get a new perspective to see things, which makes the conflict seem easier to solve. In serious situations, we tend to get offended easily, but the humor makes us less defensive, thus minimizing conflicts.

## Conflict Resolution and Anger Issues

Anger makes us do and say things that we regret later. There are various triggering factors of anger, such as financial problems, family issues, stress, etc. People with anger issues tend to get into conflicts more often. This is why conflict resolution is needed to manage anger and resolve conflicts. By following the above-mentioned steps, one will be able to manage their anger and resolve conflicts with ease.

# 10.
# Reasons Behind Passive-Aggressiveness and Coping Mechanisms

Anger is a very normal human emotion, which has been complicated by human beings themselves. More than often, anger has directly been linked to aggressiveness and violence, which in turn made us humans to believe that anger is a bad emotion and is not acceptable in society. This leads to many of us repressing the feeling of anger, which in turn slips out through passive-aggressiveness.

## What Is Passive Aggressiveness?

One of the most troublesome behavior, not just for others but for the people themselves, is passive-aggressiveness. So, what exactly does this mean to be passive-aggressive?

This is a behavior where a person expresses anger through indirect means. Normal people acknowledge the feeling of anger or frustration and eventually channels it out through words or actions. However, this is not the case with people who are passive-aggressive. Such people fail to acknowledge the particular emotion of anger, or even if they do, they consciously suppress the emotion and do not let that emotion out of them.

They suppress their emotion once, twice, and many more times. What happens then? They become a master of repressing anger. They become such experts in camouflaging their emotions that not just them but everyone around them assumes that the individual never gets angry!

A natural emotion, such as anger, can be realized and controlled, but can it be abolished? No! The contained or repressed emotion eventually seeps out, without them even realizing. Such people subconsciously do passive things that are usually rude as a method of coping with such situations that have gone beyond their control.

Unfortunately, our society is filled with people who are passive-aggressive – be it our workplace, neighborhood, or even inside our family. A person with such a passive reaction cannot be blamed completely for not rectifying their behavior, as the behavior is often not recognized by them or the people around them. This is a very complicated nature where people around them are more confused as to why a person suddenly acts the way they do.

To conclude, passive-aggressiveness is the unconscious outflow of all the negativity and anger build inside a person due to the continuous, willed suppression of emotion of betrayal, dishonesty, or any minute change in behavior which is deemed wrong by the individual. The only motive or objective of people with such passive-aggressive nature is to get even with the individual who hurt their feelings but in a sneaky manner, that is, without directly letting the antagonist of their story know that they are mad at them.

The anger evinces through various actions like being late on purpose, taunting others, saying words to enrage the person in front, confused actions, continuous brooding over a task, dissatisfaction, frustration over mere things, distant behavior towards partner or family, etc.

## Understanding the Reasons For Developing Passive-Aggressiveness

This behavior can be caused due to profuse reasons. According to some experts, this behavior is directly linked to their childhood turmoil, whereas some believe it is a choice that has grown over time. Some even link this dysfunctional behavior directly to mental state.

In reality, it can occur due to countless reasons; some of the most common reasons for such inappropriate behavior can be listed as follows:

- **Brought up in an environment filled with raging people** – It might be that as a person was growing up, his parents or relatives or neighbors always did some violent actions whenever they were angry. It might also be that as a child, whenever they did something to make their elders angry, they were subjugated to vicious acts. This might have caused them to feel scared and helpless, and now as they have grown up, they do not want people around them to be scared of them. Such individuals believe that the outcome of rage is always disastrous. They do not want to be the problematic one in the room, or they do not want to be seen the way they saw their relatives when they were enraged.

Hence, they are continuously repressing their anger by themselves on purpose cause they are also scared that the outcome of their anger is going to be nasty and violent. Psychologically, the emotion needs to be expressed, but they do not want to let it out as they are scared, which then results in them saying something or doing something to enrage anyone in front of them. All they are trying to do here is let the emotion out vicariously.

If the person in front of them is enraged and outbursts, they then feel a sense of relief. As if it was they who outbursted and got relieved of the heaviness of anger.

- **Made to have been believed that 'anger is a bad emotion'** – how often are we told: "getting angry will not solve anything"? Many a time right. Many people live with their parents and grow up in schools, where they are taught that anger is not something acceptable. As kids, some are told that anger is bad. To be a good kid, we should kill our basic emotions of anger without being told how to do it. Most of us thus chose to tuck those feelings in the back of our heads.

  To top that, the media, too, always portrays the negative aspects of anger. Cartoons also educate us that angry people are disliked by one and all, and should we want us to be likable, we need to remain calm and patient always. All these worsens the situation and messes with the young mind.

  To sum up, they are never educated about the constructive side of anger. Thus, they are made to suppress their anger, which naturally spurts out now and then as passive-aggressive behavior.

- **Passive-Aggressiveness is easier than confrontation** – Suppose a person is not keen about doing something but is repetitively told to do the same without giving them any other choice. In such a situation, they feel trapped. Now, if this is in their workplace and the needs confronting their boss, they simply chose not to. These emotions of anger do not go away, instead manifests in passive aggressiveness.

- **Choosing revenge over confrontation** – When infuriated, some of us tend to make the person, root of one's such emotion, feel the same sentiment that they did. To simply say, they seek revenge without getting caught red-handed.

Let us look at an example to understand this reason behind passive-aggressiveness properly. Suppose Mr. A works hard but is not acknowledged or given due importance. He sees people less deserving than him (according to him) prospering quicker than him. He holds his boss responsible for that. Now Mr. A is furious and wants his boss to feel the same pain and helplessness that he felt. But he cannot do anything directly since it is his boss, any mistake and it might cost him his job.

Now, what does Mr. A do? A takes up an extremely vital task in their project and starts working on it alone. In the last 2- 3 days, he calls for sick leave. The work gets slacked, and now the boss is questioned and denied promotion for the year for not being able to get the project finished on time.

Revenge served while also not getting caught in the act. This is very common in the workplace until caught since this is the easy way out of the situation with satisfaction.

- **Hunger for Power** – Passive-Aggressiveness includes brushing off any sort of feeling of anger. This presents them as the wise person to the world. This lets them play the victim card. They usually cut direct communication with the person whom they want to teach a lesson to or narrate the story portraying themselves as the victim to mutual co-workers or friends who might go and confront the other persons. This act puts the other person in a tough spot by sending them on a guilt trip. The other person starts doubting themself and feels responsible.

This gives a sense of power to the person incorporating this behavior as they get to be the puppeteer.

- **Not wanting to deal with drama** – Not everyone who exercises such behaviors is by default passive-aggressive. Some chose to occasionally act that way.

  Suppose a man is tired of week-long work and has decided to spend the weekend lazily at home, but the family constantly pressurizes him to go to the market or some other place for some work. They want their day to be peaceful as well; refusal to go outside and finish the work might bring in some unnecessary troubles. So now they deliberately become passive-aggressive. They constantly delay the trip by making silly excuses till the end.

  Thanks to this behavior, their goal is achieved by avoiding any drama.

- **The lack of practice of assertiveness** – Kids are no experts when it comes to expressing any human emotion. They need to be guided. Asserting or communicating the problems or causes of dissatisfaction is a bold move. It is more like a pearl of wisdom that needs to be instilled in kids. However, many a time, this topic of channeling anger constructively or asserting them directly gets missed by our elder.

  This results in a lack of the skill of assertion. Since the skill is missing, those individuals grow up without even knowing what to do with all the anger-filled within. They thus chose to stay silent on the matter, and the trapped heat within flows out through indirect actions.

This dysfunctional behavior can also be a cause of some direct effects of mental health like depression or anxiety disorder, substance disorder, or even disorder of personality. If so, then it is best to seek the help of a therapist.

## Why is it Important to Let Go of This Behavior or Pattern?

Passive aggressiveness can be a convenient way of getting the proper reactions from the other people and an easier way of dealing with the emotion, but only for the short term. In the long run, this is as bad as physical violence. Such behavior is mental abuse to the person facing it. In the short term, it may also seem more convenient since it requires less courage and gets the job done.

An unchecked behavior may cause constant troubles in the workplace, tensions, and distance in relationships, which may even lead to breaking up. When the partner is constantly subjected to such behavior, they are mentally abused. They feel confused and loses faith in the person, and get sick of the situation. Even if the partner realizes the root of the behavior and tries to educate them on the matter, they get trapped in the vicious cycle of the partner's denial and them getting subjected to the same behavior again. Thus, the only option left with them is to walk out of the relationship.

Not just that, denial of the feeling of anger and resorting to this behavior for a long period can cause self-harm. Bottling up such strong emotions will only make them more and more anxious, confused and eventually lead to depression. Thus, the best thing to do is to work on this behavior and conquer it to maintain a healthy flow of life.

## Various Coping Mechanisms to Deal with Passive-Aggressiveness

Most people are either passive-aggressive themselves or know at least one person who is passive-aggressive. The trouble here is that people fail to realize this dysfunctional behavior since it has become such a common phenomenon. Everyone acts in such a way or resorts to this behavior to deal with some uncalled-for situation, at least once in their lifetime, and is perfectly fine. But if this behavior becomes a constant habit or lifestyle - it needs to get rectified.

- So, the first step towards coping with this behavior is to recognize the behavior. If someone notifies you about that behavior directly or if someone tells you that you behave differently at times or if you can feel that you are a prisoner of this vicious behavior, acknowledge it.

- The major reason for such behavior is the fear of confronting someone directly! So, if you are someone who is caught up in it, try to address your issues openly without fear of judgment. You might feel like speaking the truth can break someone's heart or create a bad image of you and hence will want to stick to an indirect flow of anger. But you must realize that such behavior does not solve any problem or keep you in the good books of everyone. It only causes more chaos and attracts resentment of others towards you. So, try and be more assertive. Communicate, and you will learn that problems are solved within minutes.

- People with this behavior issue often tends to taunt others or sarcastically points to other mistakes. They also indirectly address the problem to the person. Thus, another method of coping with this is to try and incorporate more 'I's in their sentences, like, I do not like you talking to me in that way, or I get mad when you speak rudely.

- Try and work on your communication skills. The better the communication skill, the easier it will be to confront the person causing you distress.

The major challenge in coping with passive-aggressiveness is to come to terms with one's anger. Once a person can do that, they can work on this behavior and get over with it. If working on the issue by themselves is not of much help, then it is always a good option to seek therapy.

## How to Deal With a Passive-Aggressive Person?

Dealing with a passive-aggressive friend, partner, co-worker, or family member can be really frustrating and tiresome. They will constantly try to impose a feeling of guilt in you and make your life miserable in the process. Hence, properly dealing with such people is necessary. Here are a few tips on how to deal with a passive-aggressive person –

## Tip 1

If you feel like one of your family members or colleagues is exercising passive-aggressiveness, then help them realize it by addressing the problem. Address them the issues that they are creating.

## Tip 2

If you know someone who is behaving in this manner, be direct to them. Do not get caught up in their mind games. Be assertive to them, then and there itself. Do not wait for long. If you see them behaving awkwardly or rudely, directly ask them as to what is wrong and assure them that it is okay to let out the emotion of anger.

## Tip 3

Another way of dealing with people with passive-aggressiveness is to sit and talk to them. They need to be told and made to understand that anger is not a bad emotion at all. They should be made to understand that anger is a basic emotion that is just very strong and needs to be a little controlled. Anger needs an appropriate way of being expressed in keeping things from getting ugly.

## Tip 4

If the person is not willing to let go of this behavior and continues inflicting emotional abuse on you through their passive-aggressiveness, then the best thing is to avoid them. If you give in to their tricks, they will enrage you even more through their words or actions. Thus, the best thing to do is to avoid them. If you are in a relationship with such an individual, then you should perhaps take a stand and walk away from them.

# Conclusion

Thank you for making it through to the end of *The Anger Management Workbook*, let's hope it was informative and able to provide you with all of the tools you need to achieve your goals, whatever they may be.

Any habit is hard to break, be it anger or anything else but even then, you have to keep trying to be successful. If you want to come out as a better person after a month or so, follow every step that has been mentioned in this book. At times, it might even seem like an impossible task to break through your anger and bring it under your control, but you cannot lose hope. We feel this way because living with your anger is much easier than dealing with it.

Make small changes every day – meditate, socialize with people who make you feel good and positive, think positively, have your own affirmations, and so on. At present, these might seem to be insignificant and not bring much of a difference, but in the long run, this is what is going to help you deal with your anger. Remember that Rome was not built in a day, and you cannot manage your anger overnight. So, keep at it, and after a while, you will not have to think about your anger issues again.

Finally, if you found this book useful in any way, a review on Amazon is always appreciated!

www.ingramcontent.com/pod-product-compliance
Lightning Source LLC
Chambersburg PA
CBHW070658220526
45466CB00001B/483